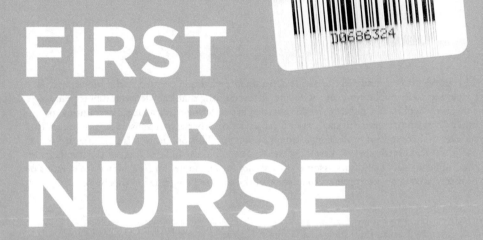

FIRST YEAR NURSE

WISDOM, WARNINGS, AND WHAT I WISH I'D KNOWN
MY FIRST 100 DAYS ON THE JOB

Edited by Barbara Arnoldussen, RN, MBA • Fourth Edition

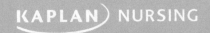
KAPLAN) NURSING

© by 2016 Kaplan Inc.

Published by Kaplan Publishing, a division of Kaplan, Inc.
750 Third Avenue
New York, NY 10017

10   9   8   7   6   5   4   3   2   1

ISBN-13: 978-1-5062-2919-5

Contents

Acknowledgments

Dedicated to my mother, Barbara A. Rudolph, RN, my favorite new nurse.

I acknowledge the excellent editorial assistance of Helena Santini. The encouragement of my husband, Tom, and the support of my family and friends were critical to accomplishing this exciting project.

A heartfelt thanks to the hundreds of nurses across the country who shared their genuine feelings and solid advice to nurture new nurses. Great teamwork!

The publisher would like to thank Judie Hogan and Karen Lilyquist for their contributions to this project.

Introduction

You are about to embark on the journey of a lifetime. You think that nursing school has prepared you for what lies ahead . . . until you begin your first job and are flooded with a huge patient load, more charting than you can finish, and multiple questions from family members, each requiring an immediate answer (that you don't have!). You need to get a handle on the situation and get oriented before you start to feel disoriented.

How can you calm the fast pace of your beating heart (or in professional diagnostic terms, your "situational tachycardia")? Don't worry, this book is here to help. It's filled with quotes and advice from several hundred nurses who have been there and done that . . . and now want to make the journey easier for you.

Packed with everything from down-to-earth humor ("There's nothing like eating popcorn from an unused bedpan!") to frank insights about maintaining motivation on the job ("Work with your heart. Every chance to learn, love, and be compassionate is a moment well spent") while including practical tips ("A good pair of bandage scissors will last a lifetime"), this book is designed to help you survive—and even thrive—during your first 100 days as a new nurse.

True to their mission of nurturing others, the nurses who contributed to this book want to help you up, over, and around the hurdles that they themselves faced. They want to make your beginning steps more confident so that you can stride with ease.

Welcome to the ranks.

CHAPTER 1

The Reality Check

"Nursing school definitely did not prepare me for all the poop I cleaned up in my first hundred days as a nurse."

–Intensive care unit nurse, Lynchburg, VA

Congratulations! You are about to make the world's most rewarding profession not just your job but your career. It is a lifelong journey like no other.

On the pages that follow, the Voices of Experience will weigh in on why they became nurses. More likely than not, you will hear some of your thoughts echoed in theirs. In turn, you will be given a heads-up as they discuss some of the surprises that come with the territory. Even though the dream has finally come true, there are going to be difficult days. The best thing is to be prepared. So read on to find out just what those reasons for nursing are, and to learn about some of the challenges that await.

MIND THE GAP

From one nurse to another, you should know a well-kept secret about nursing—there's a bigger gap than you think between nursing school and the "real world." While you'll find nursing to be a meaningful and worthwhile profession, every experienced nurse will tell you that you're in for some eye-opening surprises at the beginning . . . some good, some not.

Wondering what those surprises could be? In this chapter, seasoned nurses describe the surprises they found, so that you'll step onto the job prepared for the unexpected.

SCHOOL DAZE

"*Nothing was done like I was taught in school. Things are dictated by the Policy & Procedures manual created by the institution where you're working—so know your P&P!*"

   –OB-GYN nurse, St. Louis, MO

"*Simple things not learned in nursing school seemed complex and difficult until mastered. Every night when I came home from work I had to study about words, illnesses, and tests that I had never heard of.*"

   –Telemetry nurse, Kunkletown, PA

"*Because the material you learn in nursing school is so broad, if you are going into a focused area at your new job, it helps to relearn the material specific to that job before you start.*"

   –Neonatal intensive care unit nurse, Atlanta, GA

"It was a lot more liberating than nursing school—there was more freedom to practice your knowledge in a real setting."

–Emergency department nurse, Santa Clarita, CA

LEARNING AT THE SPEED OF LIGHT

"The first hundred days were scary, but a good opportunity to learn new things by being patient, asking lots of questions, and doing hands-on training."

–OB-GYN nurse, Olathe, KS

"I was really surprised at how much I didn't know. The best thing that I ever did was to accept my limited knowledge base and let the more experienced nurses guide me."

–Pediatric nurse, Chicago, IL

"I learned that you can't do everything by the book and you have to expect to make mistakes."

–Intensive care unit nurse, Franklin, OH

"Be ready to let go of the false belief that you must 'know everything' in order to be a good nurse. It will all come together. The imposter syndrome, while rampant among new nurses, doesn't serve us well!"

–Geriatric nurse, Gaston, OR

PRESSURE

"My orientation was fast and furious."

–Hospital staff nurse, Charleston, SC

"The most difficult adjustment has been learning to practice the art of caring and the science of nursing in the task-oriented, efficiency-driven environment. My greatest disappointment and frustrations come when the patient most needs my presence, but my assignments allow for three to five minutes with her."

–Long-term care nurse, Gaston, OR

"Time management and prioritizing were even more important and crucial than I imagined as a student. I had a full load of very sick patients who all needed tons of medications and treatments."

–Pediatric nurse, El Cerrito, CA

ORGANIZATION

"I don't think I realized how much a nurse was truly responsible for. We are the ones who keep everyone coordinated. Everyone depends on you to get 'it' done—no matter what 'it' might be!"

–Intensive care unit nurse, Parkton, MD

"In the first hundred days you learn that nursing is not all patient care. There's a ton of paperwork to be done as well."

–Telemetry nurse, Brick, NJ

"My first hundred days was all about the process of how to get things done. All it takes is one glitch in the process to slow your shift to a screeching halt. You realize there are multiple ways to accomplish any task."

–Orthopedic nurse, Seabrook, TX

WORKING ON THE HEALTH-CARE TEAM

"Not all nurses remember what it was like to be a new nurse. If they had remembered, it would not have been 'baptism by fire.'"

–Surgical nurse, Carversville, PA

"Most nurses were actually very supportive and informative despite rumors of the opposite, but there were still a few that weren't. Watch out for those few!"

–Emergency department nurse, Hagerstown, MD

"I wasn't prepared for the range of personalities of the doctors and nurses I was working with. You have to quickly adapt to each personality over the course of the day."

–Surgical nurse, Des Plaines, IL

PATIENTS AND PATIENCE

"*In some ways, patient care was easier than it was in nursing school because my instructors weren't breathing down my neck. However, in other ways it was harder because I was on my own.*"

–Surgical nurse, Ashland, KY

"*There is so much you didn't learn in school, especially the actual meaning of curing; It's something you have within you, not something you learned in Caring 101.*"

–Orthopedic nurse, Winona, MN

"*As an RN you are dealing with the different lifestyles of patients and their family members. One really has to be tolerant of others.*"

–Oncology nurse, St. Paul, MN

"You need to have a strong sense of yourself, so that you know what you can give to patients and where you may need guidance or assistance."

–Pediatric nurse, Baltimore, MD

RESPONSIBILITY FOR LIVES

"Patients can crash on you in seconds. No two days are ever the same."

–Emergency department nurse, Berlin, NJ

"I never thought that I would be taking care of eight patients at a time who were each extremely sick. . . . It was really scary."

–Surgical nurse, Barnesville, GA

"My first patient coded on the O.R. table and did not survive. Realizing the patient's life is dependent upon what you do, and even what you don't do, is sobering."

–Operating room nurse, Lynchburg, VA

A RANGE OF EMOTIONS

"I never would have guessed how emotional it is to be a new nurse. In one day I would feel extremely proud of myself, disappointed in myself, angry, sad, stressed, or even all of these at once."

–Cardiac intensive care unit nurse, Columbia, MD

"It was everything I thought it would be and more: hectic, exhausting, and rewarding all at the same time."

–Home-care nurse, Cerritos, CA

"I learned and saw more in my first hundred days than I ever thought I would see in my entire career. It was overwhelming but exhilarating."

–Medical telemetry nurse, Piedmont, CA

If you think all of that is a lot to deal with, don't worry! Starting with the next chapter, this book will give you all the info you need to travel comfortably through uncharted territory and master each challenge you come across. Chapter 2 deals specifically with preparing yourself before you even begin your first job.

Starting Off on the Right Foot

"Make sure you have a nice comfy pair of shoes—there are many miles to be walked."

—Emergency department nurse, Egg Harbor Township, NJ

Your choice of where to accept your first nursing job will set the stage for the rest of your career. Rather than feeling alone with the enormity of this decision, know that you are in good company—experienced nurses want to help you get the information you need to choose a job and give you practical advice on how to begin that job with confidence.

This chapter will aid with finding a job, determining what questions to ask about potential positions, and rating the possibilities. It will also describe some tools of the trade that will make your workday easier. Remember: The pathway to success starts even before your first day on the job!

EXPLORE JOB CHARACTERISTICS

One of the best ways to know if a nursing position is the right fit for you is to find out as much about it as you can in advance! That way, you head off any surprises and will be well informed (and therefore more relaxed) during your first hundred days on the job. Here are some questions to ask before you accept a job offer:

QUESTIONS FOR THE EMPLOYMENT OFFICE

- Do you have a new-graduate orientation program? How long does it last, and how is it combined with regular work hours?
- Will a preceptor or a mentor be assigned for an introductory period? How long will that last?

- How much paid time off do you allow for attendance at training and continuing education courses?
- Do you reimburse tuition costs for higher education courses?
- What would you say are the top two or three qualities of the most successful nurses currently working here?
- Do you have a system of merit-based raises, or are there pay increases for length of service?

QUESTIONS FOR THE CLINICAL TEAM

- How many other nurses work in that capacity, and are some of them recent grads?
- Are there any choices about shift length or start time?
- At what point do you pay overtime or differential pay?
- Would I be required to rotate to other shifts or float to other units?
- Will I have to be on call? If yes, how often?
- Are there opportunities for increased responsibility later on in the position?
- What is the staffing ratio of nurses to patients?

RECOGNIZING A JEWEL OF A JOB

The characteristics of the first organization that you choose to join are crucial to your eventual career success and satisfaction. Here's a checklist of choices to help you identify the best of what's out there:

- Room to grow professionally
- Colleagues working together as a team
- Availability of role model or mentor
- Ongoing educational resources
- Atmosphere that welcomes input and questions
- Policies and procedures that are clear and consistent
- Appreciation of individual talents
- Variety of tasks and challenges

SCOPE OUT THE SCENE

"*Make sure they give you a detailed job description. Get as much information on what duties you will be performing prior to taking the job to make sure you are comfortable with the expectations.*"

–**Pediatric nurse, Danville, IL**

"*Talk to the nurses on the floor you will be working on. The nurses are the floor and will give the new grad more insight into how the floor is run.*"

–**Cardiology nurse, Morristown, NJ**

> "*During the interview with the nurse recruiter, you should ask about the turnover rate on the unit you are going to work. If they have frequent postings, try to find out why the turnover rate is so high.*"
>
> **–Rehabilitation nurse, Bridgeport, NJ**

> "*Take your own tour of the area. Check out the people you will be working with and see if your personality 'fits' in the work environment you are seeking to enter.*"
>
> **–Rehabilitation nurse, Rancho Sante Fe, CA**

SHARE AND SHADOW

Once you've chosen a place to work, it never hurts to get yourself situated before your first day. Experienced nurses advise the following:

"*Shadowing is a wonderful thing. Shadow a nurse who works on the floor where you are going to start your new job for four hours (or even eight hours if you have the time), just to get a feel for what is in store for you.*"

–**Medical telemetry nurse, Kunkletown, PA**

"*I would definitely recommend a 'share day' on the unit of choice, to determine if the specialty is all that you thought it would be, rather than get into it because of first impressions as an outsider looking in.*"

–**OB-GYN nurse, Baltimore, MD**

GIVE ME AN "S"

Once you've explored what your new work environment will be like, you'll also want to be prepared with needed supplies. The majority of nurses in a wide range of fields agree that four items that start with the letter "S" are the most useful professional equipment for new nurses. Here are the winners:

Shoes: *"Buy the most comfortable shoes you can afford to buy, and remember to replace them often."*

   –Oncology nurse, Frederick, MD

Stethoscopes: *"Listening to breath sounds is a skill, and having a good stethoscope will help."*

   –Intensive care unit nurse, Franklin, OH

Scrubs: *"Get a scrub jacket with lots of pockets."*

   –OB-GYN nurse, Baltimore, MD

Scissors: "*A good pair of bandage scissors will last a lifetime.*"
–Medical-surgical nurse, Louann, AR

THE FEET COME FIRST!

What's the number-one most important tool for nurses? Shoes, of course! Nurses find that being on their toes all day translates into a need to ensure that their feet are well supported. You don't need to introduce white orthopedic shoes into your wardrobe, but whether you buy clogs or lace-ups, you need to pay particular attention to comfort. Check out the characteristics of each part of the shoe:

- **Broad toe box**—your toes should be able to spread out naturally. Toes are vital in maintaining your balance.
- **Deep heel cup**—to hold your protective tissue firmly in place. On hard surfaces, your own natural cushioning is stressed.

- **Neutral or unelevated heel**—this basically allows all the bones in your feet to share the burden of supporting the weight of your entire body.
- **Lightweight, shock-absorbing sole**—the 26 bones, more than 100 ligaments, and 19 muscles of the foot will appreciate it.
- **Firm arch support**—this prevents the fatigue, pain, and stiffness in your feet, legs, and lower back that can be symptoms of fallen arches.

PUTTING YOUR BEST FOOT FORWARD

Here are a few more items that experienced nurses swear by to help ease the burden on their feet:

"Compression stockings!"
   –Long-term-care nurse, Gaston, OR

"A foot massager!"
   –Emergency department nurse, Brick, NJ

"A pedometer . . . to remind everyone else just how much you're on the move at work!"

–Medical telemetry nurse, Rock Valley, IA

YOU GOTTA HAVE HEART . . . SOUNDS

Enough about feet and legs! How about using your ears? Having your own stethoscope can save you search-and-locate time and can be more comfortable. Consider these features:

Earplugs

- Your ears have a unique shape, so actually try out different models. Know what the return policy is.
- Check out the firmness and size of each earplug and headset angle. Make sure you are comfortable with the fit and weight.

Tube Length

- The longer the tube, the more sound is lost.
- With a shorter tube, you get better sound transmission, but you might have to move into a difficult-to-hold body position.

Tube Design

- Single lumen—sound moves through the tube until the tube diverges to reach each ear. This is the sleeker of the two designs.
- Two tubes—one tube leads to your right ear, and one to you left. This type usually offers better sound transmission.

The Head (The Part Placed on the Patient)

- Traditional ones have the diaphragm (for high-pitched sounds) and a bell (for low-pitched sounds). Some designs combine them into a single head.

Tip!

Your final decision will balance the factors of fit, price, and ease of hearing sounds in light of your clinical tasks.

HANDY REFERENCES

Without a doubt you will need to record many patient-care details over the course of your workday. However, making cryptic notes on the palm of your hand or on scraps of paper is not a good way to record information.

Smartphones, tablets, and other handheld devices are currently being used to record and provide information useful for understanding drug administration, lab test results, care planning, patient education, and medical terminology. You can access medical programs through online resources or via an app on your smartphone or tablet. Some of the most popular software products for nurses are the following:

AANC Bedside: *http://www.aacn.org/wd/products/content/aacn-bedside. pcms?menu=products*

AllNurses.com (nursing social network)

Ebscohost Informational Resource: *https://www.ebscohost.com/nursing/products/nursing-reference-center*

Epocrates: *http://www.epocrates.com/products/features*

Johns Hopkins Antibiotic Guide: *http://www.unboundmedicine.com/products/johns_hopkins_abx_guide*

Medscape: *http://reference.medscape.com/*

Nursing Essentials (app)

Pepid: *http://www.pepid.com/medical-apps/*

Taber's Medical Dictionary: *http://www.unboundmedicine.com/products/tabers_medical_dictionary*

UpToDate: *http://www.uptodate.com/home*

FACT REMINDERS

And for the less technologically inclined, here are some suggestions from nurses on items to help record critical information:

"A pocket clipboard with a calculator for calculating drug dosages."

–Hospital staff nurse, Homer, MI

"Small information cards, the kind that can hold tons of information and fit in your pocket for easy access. They're also good to tape on the inside or back of a clipboard for quick reference."

–OB-GYN nurse, St. Louis, MO

"A small, easy-to-carry book with normal lab values, common drugs, advanced cardiac life-saving steps, and disease processes in it. You can find many of these online."

–Hospital staff nurse, Virginia Beach, VA

TOP FIVE GIFT SUGGESTIONS FOR A NEW NURSE

(Feel free to leave the book open to this page for all to see. . . .)

"A waterproof watch. It will be used constantly! Even if you already have one, a spare is always good to have."

–Pediatric nurse, Baltimore, MD

"A school-related nursing pin. It is something to be proud of and a reminder of how hard you worked to get there. When you are having a rough day, just look at it and realize how badly you wanted to be a nurse when you were in school."

–Critical-care nurse, Norridge, IL

"Quality pens—lots of them. Nurses constantly lose them."

–Cardiology nurse, Akron, OH

"A pen that lights up for writing in the dark."

–Operating room nurse, Retsof, NY

"A supplies pouch that holds syringes, scissors, and other necessary tools of the trade."

–Critical-care nurse, Chicago, IL

BEFORE THE PLUNGE

Now you know all about choosing the right job and buying (or receiving) useful tools for a super start to your successful career. Before you dive headfirst into the job pool and step into your new work environment for the first day of orientation, seasoned nurses want you to take a deep breath....

"Make sure you have your life organized before starting that first job, because the job is so overwhelming at first that all of your extra energy is gone by the time you get to your home life—you don't have any extra to give."

–Pediatric nurse, Fort Myers, FL

"Relax/take a vacation before you start your new job. Learning new things all the time is very tiring and stressful so you'll need to rest up!"

–Operating room nurse, Retsof, NY

"Take time off between the end of your schooling and the start of a new job. Give yourself time for the excitement and anticipation to build up!"

–Medical-surgical nurse, St. Paul, MN

CONFIDENCE IS KEY!

No matter how long it seems delayed in coming, your first day of work as a new nurse will be memorable. You are opening a door to a new work environment and the start of your nursing career. Sometimes the best way to build confidence is to act confident . . . right from the start. That way, you're ready to take on whatever comes! Here's what a few nurses had to say on the subject:

"It takes a while to gain physicians' and old-school nurses' respect, but hang in there—you are all an important part of the team."

–OB-GYN nurse, Madison, WI

"Start your very first day with confidence. Unfortunately, health-care workers can sense fear, just like animals, and they prey on it. Remember, nobody was born knowing everything."

–Operating room nurse, Gilliam, MO

"Be patient with yourself. Realize that you are not going to know everything the first day or even the hundredth day of stepping on the floor. Just trust your instincts!"

–Pediatric nurse, Bedford, NY

Now you know how to choose the right job and useful equipment. You have given yourself a pep talk about confidence. Before you are assigned your first load of patients, you will want to learn about nurse-tested time management techniques. The next chapter will discuss how you can stay organized to effectively and efficiently meet the myriad demands of your new job.

CHAPTER 3

Organization 101

> "When the patients are buzzing with requests, the doctor's on
> the phone, and new admits and your coworkers are asking
> questions, you could easily forget your own name, let alone
> your next task."
>
> **–Medical-surgical nurse, Evergreen, AL**

In this chapter, nurses share with you how to have the time of your life
during work hours, by using your time well. You want to be able to meet
your patients' needs by delivering safe, quality care, but you also want to
be able to communicate with your colleagues and leave work on time with

all the required documentation complete. That's a tall order considering the endless facts to remember and the piles of paperwork to complete. However, other nurses have found organizational success—and want to share their secrets with you in this chapter.

THE BLACK-AND-WHITE OF GRAY MATTER

You will hear experienced nurses talk about their "brains" or their "cheat sheets." It's their method of writing down ticklers about what they need to accomplish that workday and at the same time have a way to record what tasks have been completed.

The key is that the "brains" have a set graphic format that does not change from day to day, and that you record information in a standard way. When designing your "brains," you can be as creative as you want. Here are some starting points. You can choose to organize by:

- **Patients in order of their room numbers or the time of their clinical visit.** Then you can go down the list and work with patients in the same order. This makes giving report easier, too.

- **Hours of the day,** so that all your 9 A.M. tasks are listed together, and so forth.

- **Clinicians.** That way, when Dr. X arrives, you will be ready to give an update on all patients.

- **Tasks, either ongoing or one time.** Then you will know all the patients who need their fluid intakes and outputs recorded throughout the day, for example, or those who need vital signs taken once a shift.

You will know you have a successful system when you can pace yourself through a full cycle of work, knowing at all times what percentage of your tasks are completed and what you still have ahead of you. Consider some ideas found on the next two pages on how nurses cloned their "brains."

RECIPES FOR BRAIN FORMATION

"*At first I had no system . . . and that slowed me down. So I asked every nurse I was paired with to show me their 'brain' and how they used it to keep track of all their patients. Every single nurse I asked told me enthusiastically about her system of organization. I created my own 'brain' based on the collection of ideas from the more experienced nurses.*"

–Orthopedic nurse, Seabrook, TX

"*I carried a three-ring binder with dividers and a pencil bag. I kept everything I needed in it. I used it to keep my notes on patients and their medication administration record close at hand. That way I had everything in one place when questions arose or a call needed to be made to a doctor.*"

–Hospital staff nurse, Lynchburg, VA

"*I have gone through my share of four-by-six note cards with scribbles about my patients on each of them. The front is split down the middle with a line. The left side of the front contains the patient's name, allergies, code status, past medical history, and current diagnosis. On the right side of the front of the card I list when meds and labs are due and also make a working list throughout the day of tasks and treatments that need to occur with a space to check when tasks are completed. On the back of the card, I list the reported assessment, working system by system (cardiovascular, respiratory, etc.).*"

–**Intensive care unit nurse, Lynchburg, VA**

THE GIVE-AND-TAKE OF REPORT

In your training, you probably practiced a communication technique basic to hospital nursing—the change-of-shift report. In order to provide for continuity of patient care in a 24/7 setting, as you came on duty, you were informed of both the routine and unique events of the previous shift. At the end of your shift, you used the same process to effectively pass the baton of care into the hands of the incoming health-care workers.

It is no coincidence that quality improvement efforts often target this transition, since the risk of a flawed communication is always present in this "handoff." See the following remarks for different methods of how experienced nurses handle their reports.

REPORT TECHNIQUES

"I record my reports the same way every single shift. This helps in finding information as well as not wasting valuable time looking for information."

–Cardiology nurse, Ellicott city, MD

" I basically had to know everything about my patient in a matter of hours, so I had to learn to skim the chart and, when taking report, always ask questions. That was something I had to get used to, just formulating the right questions to ask, so that I had the best clinical picture of my patients, system by system. "

–Medical telemetry nurse, Pico Rivera, CA

" All the info from the previous shift was in black. I added everything that happened on my shift in red. At the end of the day, I knew that everything in red was something that I should chart or give report on. "

–Hospital staff nurse, Center, TX

THE CHA-CHA OF CHARTING

Whereas the change-of-shift report is only found in health-care environments providing round-the-clock care, you will encounter some version of charting (keeping a permanent record of each patient's history) in all nursing jobs.

Just as expert dancing is based on your getting into the rhythm of the musical beat, so too does expert charting depend on your discovering what timing makes the most sense for you. Experienced nurses have a variety of approaches to share with you on the next page.

CHARTING—NOW OR LATER?

"*Always try to chart as soon as you finish with a patient. That way, you can write it down and go on to the next task with a fresh mind.*"

–Home health care nurse, McIntyre, GA

"*I have a deal with myself that I don't eat my lunch until my charting is caught up.*"

–**Hospital staff nurse, Baltimore, MD**

"*Everyone finds their own system that works for them. Mine is to do what needs to be done and chart it later. We do computer charting. Since most patients are on fetal monitors, I chart on the strip that records the baby's heartbeat and put it in the computer record when I get time.*"

–**OB-GYN nurse, Point Pleasant, WV**

"*I tried to focus on the patient and what the patient's needs were—charting was the last thing on my mind and was left for the end of the day. It was hard to see my coworkers leaving when I had so much left to do, but it was easier every day, and I was able to get a grasp on time management.*"

–**Hospital staff nurse, Fort Myers, FL**

JOB-SPECIFIC REFERENCE MATERIAL

From your first day at your new job, you will be gathering a lot of general information about how to function in that environment. You can assemble your own how-to guide, resource list, or visual aids. The key is to be ready to capture all the facts in one place as soon as you recognize that you might need them in the future. Examples of useful information include:

- Telephone and pager numbers to reach physicians during regular hours
- The after-hours on-call system procedures
- Telephone extensions of ancillary departments, with brief notes on which lab test or x-ray they handle and their hours
- Turnaround times for usual lab results
- Vendors of often-prescribed equipment
- Abbreviations and acronyms approved for use, since they differ from facility to facility
- Notes about specialized medications and treatments for your patient population

The next few pages cover some more time-saving tips from nurses. Stay calm, don't panic, and do one thing at a time. Learn from your mistakes.

A LIBRARY OF IDEAS

"*I made my own book of how to make arrangements for specialists' consultations and how often-ordered tests are scheduled. It's a resource guide to my institution (very job-specific).*"

–**Oncology nurse, Winnsboro, TX**

"*I kept a planner where I wrote all my appointments and my work schedule. I also wrote out weekly and monthly goals.*"

–**Hospital staff nurse, San Francisco, CA**

"*I kept flashcards. I was learning at an exponential rate, and it was impossible to remember everything. In truth, learning takes time, so I tried to decrease the time it took by writing things down so I wouldn't have to ask the same questions. For a while it didn't seem like it was working but over time it definitely paid off. Now, I rarely refer to my flashcards, but I wouldn't dare throw them away.*"

–Pediatric nurse, El Cerrito, CA

"*It's easier to get a handle on the routine day-to-day activities once you know what you're doing. But the thing about nursing is that it's highly unpredictable—and nurses have to learn to adjust at a moment's notice.*"

–Dermatology nurse, Chicago, IL

PRACTICAL PRIORITIZATION

"*I had to learn that some things can wait. Then I had to learn to trust my judgment on what could wait.*"

–**Critical-care nurse, Fayetteville, NC**

"*You have to know which of your patients are the sickest. They need your immediate attention. Try to get as many things done as you can when you enter someone's room (i.e., do the IV, lab work, medications, etc., all at the same time). It will save you a lot of time running back and forth from the nurses' station to the patient's room.*"

–**Emergency department nurse, Egg Harbor Township, NJ**

"*Oriented with six different nurses the first six weeks of employment. I observed their routines and tried them myself, to see which worked best.*"

–**Rehabilitation nurse, Bridgeport, NJ**

"I prepare my morning meds. Then I go to each of my patients' rooms and introduce myself and ask if they are in pain (so I can bring in pain medication right away or with their morning meds)."

–Orthopedic nurse, Waterford Works, NJ

STAYING FLEXIBLE

"I've learned that planning out a day in nursing only makes you angry because you have to go with the flow and prioritize as things are presented to you."

–Orthopedic nurse, Winona, MN

"Working in an acute hospital setting brings changes in patient assignment at a moment's notice. You have to learn to go with the flow and stay ahead of the day."

–OB-GYN nurse, Fort Riley, KS

"*I worked with several different nurses since I was assigned to an operating room for two weeks at a time. It was difficult because each nurse had her own way of doing things. For instance, when I would prep an extremity, the nurse I was working with would say, 'Don't do it like that, do it like this.' I learned to adapt to whom I was working with at the time.*"

   –Operating room nurse, Ontario, CA

JUST-IN-TIME LEARNING

"*I check the surgery schedule a day ahead, so I can find out as much as possible about a diagnosis or procedure happening the next day.*"

   –Operating room nurse, Retsof, NY

"I make a to-do list every night after I've finished my charting and my medication administration record sheet."

–Hospital staff nurse, Knoxville, TN

"Understand that nursing is always a learning process. If you are dealing with a new drug or a new piece of equipment, research what you are dealing with."

–Hospital staff nurse, Columbus, OH

AVOIDING OVERLOAD

"Think hourly, but also remember the big picture."

–Critical-care nurse, Fairfield, CT

"If you start to feel unorganized, take a break, sit down, and make a timetable for what has to be done."

   –Oncology nurse, Orlando, FL

"It was very difficult to adjust because I had to find what worked for me. . . . I had to find the routine that allowed me to be an advocate, an educator, a listener, a learner, and a team player. So if I needed help, I asked for it."

   –Pediatric nurse, Fairfax Station, VA

"If you ever get overwhelmed, take time out to regroup. Do not let the environment control you; you can control the environment."

   –Emergency department nurse, Hagerstown, MD

Now that you have a toolbox of techniques to get better organized, you are ready to look at the many facets of your new job from another point of view. It took seasoned nurses many years to learn about the essence of their healing roles from the patients and families they cared for. They don't want you to have to wait as long . . . so read Chapter 4 to enjoy their practical insights about your new career.

The Many Sides to Patient Care

> "*I remember the first time a patient squeezed my hand, looked into my eyes, and said, 'Thank you.' At that moment I knew that I was in the right profession. I've learned from my patients that you only have to give them five minutes of your time to make a difference, in their lives and in your own.*"
>
> **–Orthopedic nurse, Winona, MN**

As you saw in the last chapter, there's so much organizing to be done during the workday that it's easy to forget about your number-one role as a nurse: CAREgiver. Your own unique personality and nurturing behavior contribute greatly to the healing environment—probably more than you realize. Read on to find out what experienced nurses learned from patients and families and how it changed their perception of nursing.

THERAPEUTIC DIALOGUE

From the time you introduce yourself to a patient to the time you say good-bye, you'll find that your words and attitude are a powerful part of the healing process. It's amazing how much conversations can contribute, whether it's to help put patients at ease, teach them how to care for themselves, or relay messages from their doctors. Here are some tips on making these discussions go as smoothly as possible:

Do:

- **Stand or sit a comfortable distance from the person to whom you are speaking.** You don't want the patient to feel as though you are intimidating or avoiding being close.
- **Maintain direct eye contact with the person to let him know you are 100 percent there and listening**—unless the patient is too threatened by direct eye contact or it obviously increases his discomfort level. Have a calm facial expression and a body posture indicating comfort and professionalism.
- **Ask clarifying questions if necessary,** and answer all questions that you are asked in an unhurried manner.

Don't:

- **Assume the patient knows what you're talking about.** Always check with her to see if she understands what you're explaining.
- **Forget to address everyone in the room.** The family members are just as anxious to hear what you have to say as the patient is.
- **Use medical terminology** that the patient and family might not understand.

LENDING AN EAR

"Take the time to listen to patients and their families. They do not always tell you the whole story or whole truth in the first minutes that you meet them."

–Emergency department nurse, Egg Harbor Township, NJ

"Most family members in any kind of health-care setting want their questions answered and somebody to help calm their fears."

–Medical-surgical nurse, Georgetown, KY

"It really doesn't matter how well you can give a shot or do a dressing change. Usually, the best medicine is a good conversation."

–Orthopedic nurse, Hallandale, FL

"*Patients know themselves better than you do sometimes. If you are passing a med and a patient says 'I wasn't taking that yesterday,' make sure you check, because maybe it is a mistake.*"

–Intensive care unit nurse, Ellicott City, MD

ASSEMBLING YOUR OWN TEACHING RESOURCES

You will educate many people in your nursing career. You will continuously encounter patients and family members who will want to learn all about the condition that has brought them into your care—and will look to you to teach them. Think about using visual aids to support your efforts from the start. You can better engage people in the learning process with pictures, diagrams, or handouts. Here's how to prepare:

Do:

- **Keep your textbooks in a place where you can refer to them as needed** (no matter how much you might want to have a bonfire with them!).

- **Collect illustrations from articles in newspapers or magazines highlighting new health discoveries.** These items are great to share with your coworkers as well as to help educate patients. Keep a folder at home, labeled "patient education." You will be surprised how many times you will delve into it over the years, as you broaden or change the scope of your professional activity.

Don't:

- **Toss all the free literature from exhibit booths at conferences or handouts from pharmaceutical companies.** Keep some current ones for your files.

- **Worry if the content of the material matches what you envision as your future career.** The important "keep" or "throw away" decision rule is: Does the item create an "Aha!" moment for you? Do you understand the concept better after reading the materials? If yes, keep them.

> **Tip!**
>
> Get a three-ring notebook binder and put a set of vinyl document covers
> on it. Now you can quickly shove material into each sleeve without
> having to punch holes in the papers each time. Add to that a cover sheet
> with numbered dividers, and after a week or two, arrange the pages by
> category. Voila! An instant reference book!

BEING A HEALTH-CARE ENCYCLOPEDIA

"*Patients and families like you to keep them informed. At this
point in their lives, this is the most important thing going on
for all of them.*"

–**Orthopedic nurse, Fridley, MN**

"*People are less anxious about what they understand. Less
anxious family members make less anxious patients.*"

–**Critical-care nurse, Fayetteville, NC**

"*I find that sometimes I do more family education than patient education. Family members are much more apprehensive and need a lot of reassurance.*"

–Intensive care unit nurse, North Highlands, CA

"*Families and patients depend on their nurses to give them more information than their doctors. They tend to be more comfortable asking their nurse what they don't understand.*"

–Emergency room nurse, Santa Clarita, CA

"*Teaching is vital. The basic survival needs—proper diet, exercise, wound care, etc.—that you may take for granted, the patient or family have no understanding of.*"

–Pediatric nurse, Fort Myers, FL

"*It's okay to not know everything. It's more important to know where to find the answers.*"

–Public health nurse, Saratoga, CA

INCREASING YOUR CULTURAL COMPETENCY

To make sure that you know how to respond effectively to the particular patient population that you serve, you might need to learn more about different cultures, lifestyles, and religions. Here are some tips on dealing with these types of situations:

Do:

● **Learn as much as you can about the backgrounds of the patients you care for, especially their health practices and nutrition habits.** One online source of information is *www.ethnomed.org*.

- **Be ready to apologize if you make a mistake that could be seen as disrespectful.** Some patients will be delighted to take the opportunity to teach you about their background.

Don't:

- **Stereotype individuals** based on the fact that they belong to a certain cultural or religious group.
- **Forget that some cultures use different substances to improve their health, ones that they do not classify as medications.** In order to avoid adverse interactions with new medications, you need to know about the herbs and other remedies that they are taking.
- **Miss the excitement** of learning a different perspective on life and health.

TREATING EACH PATIENT AS AN INDIVIDUAL

"*Some patients have interesting values, beliefs, and points of view that you could never fathom. Be respectful and kind, no matter what you do or don't agree with.*"

–Orthopedic nurse, Waterford Works, NJ

"*People have different backgrounds but the same basic needs. Caring and compassion are essential for positive patient outcomes. Additionally, a hug or a squeeze of a hand goes a long way to let your patients and families know how much you care!*"

–Critical-care nurse, Rio Rancho, NM

"*Our patients really do depend on us to give them the best possible care for their individual needs. This includes physical, emotional, mental, and spiritual needs as well as their cultural needs.*"

–Operating room nurse, Barnesville, GA

BEING A PATIENT ADVOCATE

"*Speaking up when it's needed . . . taking action when it's required . . . you must do it, not because it's easy or comfortable, but because you want to provide the best health care you can. Keep it up, for over time, you will become aware of your positive impact on people's lives. Nursing is truly being a patient's advocate when she is unable to voice her opinion in times of grief, pain, anxiety, or sadness.*"

–OB-GYN nurse, Baltimore, MD

"*I have found my role helping patients to empower themselves and get involved in their own health-care plan, ask questions, and learn strategies for maintaining their health.*"

–Neurology nurse, St. Paul, MN

"I often work with people who are voiceless because of cognitive impairment. I have been given the privilege of developing all my senses to learn from them about their needs."

–Long-term-care nurse, Gaston, OR

"Patients oftentimes are scared—jump in and help them. If they have a bunch of questions that you are unable to answer and it is late at night, encourage them to write them down so they can ask the physician in the morning."

–Recovery room nurse, Lynchburg, VA

LINKING THE PATIENT AND CLINICIAN

"I am the individual who connects the patient to the doctor and ensures his humanity isn't lost along with all the medical treatments we provide."

–Medical nurse, St. Catharine's, Ontario

"As nurses we are the MDs' eyes, ears, and nose. We have to communicate to the MDs because they aren't with the patient— we are. Also, we have to connect with the MDs when we know that things like pain control aren't being met."

–Medical-surgical nurse, Louann, AR

"Patients ask us questions about what their doctor is planning on doing because the doc didn't explain things in a way the patient or family could understand. I tell them if they don't understand what the doc is saying, then tell her that."

–OB-GYN nurse, Point Pleasant, WV

COMFORTING THE SICK

"*Every illness and disease takes its toll not only on the physical stamina of patients, but on their emotional well-being. That's where you come in, paying attention to people's psychological needs for support and care. Your nurturing actions enhance your other healing efforts in many ways, as nurses have found. You can give 100 percent all shift long; not one med, vital sign, or lab result is overlooked, not even a second stick is needed for that blood draw or IV start. But what patients find important is if you remembered to bring them that juice and blanket you promised.*"

–Orthopedic nurse, Seabrook, TX

"*Patients are worried, frightened, and need reassurance from someone. Doctors are too busy to render the 'personal touch.' You are there to give it, and they appreciate that.*"

–Emergency department nurse, Rancho Sante Fe, CA

"Families often need the nurse to validate their concerns, hear their grief, and be their hands and feet in their absence."

–Long-term-care nurse, Gaston, OR

"Our role is not only to help patients heal physically, but spiritually and emotionally. Since we are with them 12 hours a day, our attitude has to be its best."

–Critical-care nurse, Searcy, AR

"People have a better time dealing with potential loss if they know what to expect. A caring nurse can make a difficult experience much easier to handle."

–Critical-care nurse, Fayetteville, NC

BEING THERE AT CRITICAL TIMES

"*I do a lot of teaching with patients about what to expect with a new baby. They are all very glad you are there. A new baby is scary for them.*"

–OB-GYN nurse, Kansas City, MO

"*A lot of trust comes with that diploma, but just because you've earned it with your brain doesn't mean you've earned it with your heart. That comes when you've sat with a patient or a family member while they are told something devastating or while you waiting for someone to pass away, or you have to tell family members that they didn't get there in time to be with their loved one while he passed.*"

–Medical telemetry nurse, Townsend, DE

THE FACE OF HEALING

"*Nurses are the faces that the patients see most of the time during their treatment. When you are in a bad mood, it affects the patients negatively. Also, when people go to the hospital, they lose their dignity very quickly with all the staff helping change them, bathe them, and feed them.*"

–Hospital staff nurse, Ellicott City, MD

"*You are who the patients and their families see. So be seen. You are who the patients and their families talk to. So talk to them. I have worked with people who are elderly, confused, critically ill, and/or dying. And now I work with younger people having babies. Both types of clients need compassion, understanding, competence, and friendliness.*"

–OB-GYN nurse, St. Louis, MO

"Patients and families are very well aware of the nursing shortage. They see us flying up and down the hallways all day long and are amazed that we are able to get the job done. They realize that nurses are the glue that keeps things together."

–Medical telemetry nurse, Brick, NJ

NURSES DO IT ALL!

"Most patients and their families are very dependent on the nurse and request a lot of things that are not even medically related. Not only is the nurse their lifeline to the doctor, but also their secretary, teacher, housekeeper, psychologist, and nutritionist."

–Hospital staff nurse, Whispering Pines, NC

"I am not only a nurse, but a mediator, waitress, custodian, and friend."

–Medical-surgical nurse, Kansas City, MO

"No matter what you do for your patient, your interpersonal relationship and the compassion and concern you share is what she will remember. Your actions touch lives."

–OB-GYN nurse, Phoenix, AR

"Every patient has a different situation than the next patient; as a nurse, you take on so many roles to become what your patient needs at that particular moment in her life."

–Medical-surgical nurse, Lynchburg, VA

This chapter's exploration of the many roles that nurses have learned from patients and families was rewarding. But dealing with patients and families is not always positive and upbeat.

The next chapter will take you through potentially difficult situations that nurses face. Seasoned nurses want you to have the benefits of their experience so you can enter each situation with poise and understanding.

CHAPTER 5

Coping with Challenging Patients

"Difficult patients, hostile patients, manipulative patients, depressed patients, patients with pain. Every patient requires a different approach."

–Surgical nurse, Belmont, CA

During your clinical rotations in nursing school, you probably encountered at least one unsettling patient-care issue (a dying patient or a demanding relative). You probably also cared for an individual (or two) who sensed how to push your buttons . . . and then did!

During your first hundred days at your new job, you will face a wide range of challenging issues and people. Don't feel as though you have to learn how to cope all by yourself. This chapter will give you practical tips, issue by issue, so that you can handle any crisis that comes your way.

WHAT TO DO WHEN A PATIENT IS IN PAIN

Disease hurts. Surgery hurts. Even the healing process sometimes hurts. To best help the patient cope with pain:

Do:

- **Remember that pain is the "fifth vital sign."** That means that it is as important a measure of the patient's bodily functioning as the four classic vital signs of temperature, pulse, respiration, and blood pressure. Pain must be evaluated on a regular basis.

- **Use a consistent pain scale each time you assess the patient,** such as the one that asks the patient to rate her discomfort from 0 (no pain) to 10 (the worst pain imaginable).

- **Learn to recognize the silent signs of discomfort:** restlessness, irritability, or unwanted changes in a patient's vital signs, such as marked increases in pulse, respiration, or blood pressure.

Don't:

- **Hold back pain medication ordered for a terminal patient,** worrying about the tolerance and addiction potential of drugs.

- **Rely solely on chemical means of relieving pain;** consider using environmental measures such as adding soothing music or physical actions, such as bringing another pillow or blanket or helping change the body position.

- **Forget to document the patient's response to the medication or other interventions.** The next nurse needs to know what worked, and what didn't provide sufficient pain relief.

PROVIDING PAIN RELIEF

"*At first I had difficulty knowing how to determine what is too much or too little to keep the patient comfortable. Now I look for subtle signs from the patient that tell me he is not comfortable (moans, grimaces, or change in breathing).*"

–Hospital staff nurse, Eden Prairie, MN

"*Many MDs are very conservative with pain meds, and trying to convince them that their patient is in pain and needs meds can be quite a challenge. Now I point out to them that pain, together with the stress hormones caused by it, can severely impact wound healing, increase incidence of infections, and lengthen hospital stays.*"

–Intensive care unit nurse, San Diego, CA

"*Pain issues were overwhelming when I didn't know how to draw up medications and administer them correctly. Now that I am familiar with the administration of specific medications, I see this as a way I can help my patients.*"

–**Medical-surgical nurse, St. Paul, MN**

HOW TO DEAL WITH COMPLAINTS

You just might find that you'll often function as a one-person complaint department for patients and families. And unfortunately, you will have to listen to each and every complaint and resolve the problem! Here are some useful techniques for dealing with the situation:

Do:

- **Ask questions.** It will give you a better idea of what went wrong, how, and what the follow-up course of action should be.

- **Offer to refer clinical issues to the physician promptly.**
- **Have a list handy of how to contact other resources** that handle specific nonclinical complaints, such as the admission, billing, or insurance offices.

Don't:

- **Get defensive or impatient.** This will only escalate the friction between the patient and yourself.
- **Forget to listen with care.** Sometimes people need to just be heard or express their frustration.
- **Omit the important step of documenting the interaction and the interventions that you took on behalf of the patient.** If someone else needs to follow up later, they can know about your initial work and not repeat or counteract your efforts.

DEALING WITH UNHAPPY PATIENTS

"Unhappy, disgruntled, irate patients were a challenge at first, but now I just do my best to not personalize their anger."

–Pediatric nurse, Chula Vista, CA

"*Working with patients who felt like they had not gotten appropriate care from the nurse on the shift before mine was a challenge to me. I handle this type of challenge by acknowledging the patient's frustration and asking what I can do to make his stay better.*"

   –Hospital staff nurse, Knoxville, TN

"*I try to listen to complaints with an empathetic ear and help patients talk through their frustrations. I also try to remember that being in a hospital means someone is sick and is therefore in need of excellent, compassionate care.*"

   –Orthopedic nurse, Gainesville, FL

HOW TO WORK WITH NONCOMPLIANT PATIENTS

It can be an eye-opening and frustrating experience to work with patients who don't want to participate in an opportunity to better their health—especially when all you want to do is help them improve. To best handle these frustrations:

Do:

- **Recognize that making decisions about lifestyles and habits is a choice,** and you cannot make decisions for others.
- **Consider that you might not know the whole story behind the patient's decision.** Many factors might have contributed to the situation. Later on, the patient might choose to share that information with you, but don't press.
- **Give patients time to change their minds.** All it might take is for you to leave the room for a while and let the patient ponder the situation alone for him to see your point of view.

Don't:

- **Grade yourself according to how often the patients accept your advice.** Instead, rate your educational efforts according to how clear your explanation was as far as outlining the expected outcomes and necessary steps.

- **Forget to document your patient education efforts and the patient's response.** That will help the next nurse who tries to give the same input.

- **Forget that there are always ways to work around a problem.** For example, you cannot convince someone to stop smoking. You can, however, set limits on an individual's ability to smoke in your area.

GOING AGAINST THE GRAIN

"*I now realize that people have very different expectations in regards to their hospitalization. I remain respectful and involve the patient to the level that he wishes to be involved.*"

–Critical-care nurse, Norridge, IL

"Sometimes patients can be very difficult and order you around like a servant, when they are plenty capable of doing things themselves safely. In this case, the key is to be assertive, be polite, and professionally encourage them to do things for themselves."

   –Telemetry nurse, Newtown, PA

"The single most challenging issue to me as a new nurse was learning to motivate those who couldn't or wouldn't motivate themselves. Now, instead of looking at it as an obstacle to the provision of quality care, I address it as a challenge and meet it head-on. Often, simply addressing the problem with a patient is a great way to begin!"

   –Surgical nurse, Winston-Salem, NC

DISRUPTIVE AND ABUSIVE PATIENTS

Some patients might disagree with you or refuse to comply with a request—but other patients take it one step further, in the form of yelling, causing a scene, or getting physical. These are serious situations, and here's how you can cope:

Do:

- **Put limits on what is and what is not acceptable behavior** at as early a stage as you can, and you may be able to avoid an explosive situation altogether.

- **Try to de-escalate the behavior of the individual by responding quickly and calmly to the situation.** Remember to maintain a nonaggressive posture and keep a safe, nonthreatening distance between you and the patient.

- **Give the patient several options for action and, most important,** don't compromise the patient's self-esteem or dignity. Talking down to her will only make her more angry. Communicate the situation, your response, and any aftermath to the rest of the team. Make a written report if necessary. Then others will be aware of the potential for danger.

- **Rehash the situation afterward with your supervisor or teammates** to see what pointers can be learned or policies changed to better deal with such events in the future.

Don't:

- **Feel that you have to go it alone in handling the situation.** Ask for assistance from your team members well before your need for support is crucial.

- **Hesitate to call your security staff or the police in accordance with agency policy.** No one should later criticize your actions, but if they do, remember that you are responsible for your own safety and the safety of others.

SAFETY IN NUMBERS

"*Know the telephone numbers to security or the charge nurse by heart!*"

–Emergency department nurse, Broken Arrow, OK

"When we have potentially violent patients on the ward, I prioritize ensuring that there is a proper amount of staff available to keep the patients and staff safe."

–Psychiatric nurse, Greencastle, PA

"With manipulative patients, you just have to be firm and show them that you're the one in control."

–Hospital staff nurse, Long Beach, CA

"When patients get out of line, you need to be assertive and let them know that what they are doing or saying is inappropriate, and make sure you aren't doing anything or acting in any way to promote such behavior."

–Telemetry nurse, Newtown, PA

ANGER MANAGEMENT

"Find out what is bothering the angry patient; it usually isn't what he is yelling about."

–Ambulatory-care nurse, Rochester, NY

"It can be very challenging to break the ice and get angry patients to trust you. I try to make them laugh, to pull them out of their shells. Sometimes, they won't admit it, but they do feel a sense of security when they see a familiar face the next day. They might still feel angry, but they usually open up a little bit."

–Rehabilitation nurse, Bridgeport, NJ

"We forget sometimes that patients are out of their natural settings. Some patients are taking new medications they have never taken before, and new medications can trigger an adverse response. Many times antianxiety medications can help the situation."

–Cardiology nurse, Ellicott City, MD

DISRUPTIVE AND ABUSIVE FAMILIES

Sometimes patients' friends and relatives are even more difficult to deal with than the patients—especially when there are several of them and just one of you! Consider these guidelines:

Do:

- **Let the family members know that their behavior is not acceptable in the health-care environment.** Sometimes a simple reminder that patients need a quiet environment is enough to make people settle down. They might not whisper, but everyone will feel calmer.

- **Check out your environment for your own safety and that of your other patients and their visitors;** you might need support from other staff or security. Don't let a family member come between you and the doorway.

Don't:

- **Let abusive people intimidate you into letting them not follow standard policies, such as visiting hours.** If they want to argue, give them the name of the appropriate staff person and how to contact him.

- **Forget to let the next shift or future caregivers know about the details** of the problems you faced and how you dealt with them.

- **Think that you have been singled out for this negative attention.** You were in the wrong place, or presented unhappy news, or unknowingly touched an open nerve. It is not your fault, so don't feel like you're to blame.

DIFFICULT FAMILY MEMBERS

"I didn't understand the dynamics in the beginning, but now I am starting to realize that sometimes angry or bitter family members are only reacting to their own coping mechanisms in order to keep some level of sanity during a family crisis."

—Cardiology nurse, Knoxville, TN

"When patients and their families get mad at you and are rude, just let these things go in one ear and out the other."

—Emergency department nurse, Santa Clarita, CA

"Try to help angry relatives understand the health-care process. Bend over backward to resolve the situation. It makes the delivery of health care to the patient much more effective."

–Orthopedic nurse, Hallandale, FL

"Challenging at first were those families who would write down everything I did and take all issues up to the highest in command. Now I'm confident in my practice, and I document everything!"

–Critical-care nurse, Scranton, PA

"Families expect the nurse to be at bedside much more than staffing allows. They feel slighted if the nurse has to attend to other patients and duties. Several family members have demanded that a nurse be present at all times. As a result, I have found myself having to explain staffing limits and insurance payment limits much more than I ever expected."

–Long-term-care nurse, Oak Ridge, TN

" People's expectations are different from family to family. Some expect you to wait on them hand and foot. Others know you are busy and have other patients. You need to know where they are coming from and help them as best you can."

—Emergency department nurse, Osage, IA

OVERCOMING COMMUNICATION BARRIERS

Clear and direct communication with patients and families is essential to your working together with them to meet their health-care needs. You will encounter a variety of barriers: very complex clinical conditions, hearing impairments, illiterate patients, foreign languages, and cultures that discourage openness about private matters. Here are some pointers:

Do:

- **Know what resources you have available** in terms of formal interpreters and colleagues who are conversant in other languages.

- **Slowly talk the patient through the entire process.** Let him know that answering a series of questions is part of the usual care process. Ask the patient to repeat back to you your instructions for self-care, especially if they are complex. You might have to restate the steps or further explain techniques.

- **Put instructions in writing or use pictures.** Sometimes one form of communication works better than another.

Don't:

- **Nod in agreement if you don't understand what the patient or family is saying,** due to an accent or language barrier. Let them know when their message is getting across and when it is not.

- **Give up if you reach a dead end.** Be creative and think of a different approach, other words, new pictures. Consider the situation as an opportunity for you to expand your educational skills.

- **Use medical jargon in explaining the treatment planned for the patient.** Using abbreviations or shorthand references might produce unnecessary anxiety.

TALK THE TALK

"*In a community health setting, language barriers are difficult. We use interpreters, and we try to learn some of the common second languages, like Spanish.*"

–Public health nurse, Danville, IL

"*Communicating with some patients can be difficult and can make or break your day. While it may require extra work, what these patients really need is some extra attention. The natural tendency is to spend as little time as possible in their rooms. Don't do that. If you take the time to work with them, at the end of the day, they are much more comfortable and happy.*"

–Pediatric nurse, Chicago, IL

HELPING SUBSTANCE ABUSERS

People who are ill or injured can also have drug or alcohol problems. Sometimes that's the main reason for their seeking help; more often it is a background situation. Either way, you will want to know effective ways to help them:

Do:

- **Take a careful history of legal and nonlegal drugs,** so that you can predict how the medications and procedures planned for the patient will affect her.

- **Listen to staff members who have had many years of successfully dealing with substance abusers.** Follow their lead even if it seems harsh at first. Then at another time ask them how they came to use that approach.

- **Attend continuing education courses designed to expand the repertoire of nurses who work with substance abusers on a regular basis,** even if your exposure is episodic. You will gain a useful fund of knowledge.

Don't:

- **Label the patient by the addiction when talking to your teammates.**
  The person should not be called "the heroin user" if that individual has
  come into treatment for an unrelated condition.

- **Bring your own moral philosophy into play** when dealing with the
  patient. You are not there to judge, but to provide care.

- **Forget that family members are part of the care and recovery picture.**
  Let them know of sources of community support, such as Al-Anon, if
  they are willing to seek help for themselves. If you can, make the referral
  as specific as possible as to hours and location for the meetings.

ADDICTION ADDS UP

"*When it comes to dealing with people who are under the
influence of either drugs or alcohol, you are dealing not only
with a difficult patient, but also with law enforcement in many
cases. What you can bring to the situation is to know more
about what resources are available for them.*"

–Emergency department nurse, Osage, IA

"I work with moms who have used drugs during pregnancy, and their babies also test positive for drugs. As a nurse, you have to treat everyone the same, without passing judgment. The best thing to do is to offer teaching and resources to them so that they may get help."

–OB-GYN nurse, Kansas City, MO

"We get many patients who are withdrawing from alcohol or drugs. I had to learn to remember that addiction is an illness, just like cancer or heart disease."

–Medical telemetry nurse, Townsend, DE

PATIENTS WHO ARE MENTALLY CHALLENGED

If you choose to work with patients with impaired memories and diminished intellect in either an acute or chronic health-care setting, you will find that they need special handling.

Do:

- **Request a psychiatric consult** if you feel that expertise will help the patient.
- **Review the medications ordered on a regular basis,** to check for side effects, such as confusion, being caused by the drugs.
- **Make sure that the person is getting adequate nutrition,** because malnutrition can cause an electrolyte imbalance, which in turn can trigger mental problems.

Don't:

- **Raise your voice to try to get your message across to the patient.** It is not deafness that prevents them from understanding your directions.
- **Omit the family members from participation in designing the care plan.** They know the patient and can be a wonderful source of ideas that have worked in the past or in another setting.
- **Forget to ask your coworkers for support when you need a lift or respite from a particular patient-care assignment.** Sometimes just rotating assignments is enough to give a fresh look to the workload. And don't forget to do the same for them!

PATIENTS WITH DEMENTIA

"*Alzheimer's and dementia patients are the hardest for me. I usually take a proactive approach to do as much for the patient as possible and also to ask for help.*"

   –Hospital staff nurse, Whispering Pines, NC

"*Accept demented residents as the persons they are, even if you find you will spend your whole day pacifying them with their moods. Patience is the key.*"

   –Long-term-care nurse, Martinez, CA

"*It is hard dealing with some elderly clients, because sometimes they immediately forget what it is you said. Frequent reorientation can help.*"

   –Cardiology nurse, Ellicott City, MD

HOW TO DEAL WITH DYING

Patients who are dying need to have the full range of physical-, mental-, emotional-, and spiritual-care activities available as needed to help them prepare for their death. You might be their only conduit to these resources, so you might want to consider the following approach:

Do:

- **Remember that patients have a range of emotional responses to terminal illness.** Denial, anger, bargaining ("If only I get better, I will . . ."), depression, even acceptance. These reactions are neither sequential nor universal, but it is useful to know to expect them. Then you can educate stressed patients that the negative feelings they have are normal reactions.

- **Let the patient and family members know about the phases of anticipatory grief (see the next section) and allow them to discuss their emotions about the expected demise.** Be aware of the dying person's fears, the most common of which is being left alone at the time of death. Let her know about visiting hours and if any overnight arrangements are available for friends and family members.

● **Let the patient know what you can do to make him more comfortable,** and check up on him on regular intervals, so that you can make sure the medications or other interventions, such as giving sips of water or ice chips, are effective.

Don't:

● **Forget that your nursing care can make a significant difference, even when the prognosis is grave.** In addition to pain relief, you might be able to help shortness of breath, agitation, anxiety, and depression.

ANTICIPATORY GRIEF

There is no set pattern among patients, family members, and friends when dealing with the inevitable death of a loved one. However, everyone will experience some unsettling phases. You can let them know that these are perfectly normal during the crisis:

- **Accepting the knowledge that death is inevitable.** This could engender sadness, guilt, and fear, as well as less expected effects such as poor concentration and fatigue.

- **Feeling concern for and wanting rapport with the dying person.** A frank dialogue between the caring people affected by the upcoming death can ease the suffering of all concerned. Themes of forgiveness, appreciation, and love can produce a sense of a solid, if final, linkage.

- **Rehearsing for those last few moments.** This phase concentrates on making plans for saying a final goodbye, and for making funeral arrangements. If possible, have a role in making sure that the details of the timing and privacy are optimized.

- **Imagining what the situation is going to be like after the death.** The family might envision its traditions and rituals without their loved one; the dying person might be thinking about an afterlife. Ask if they'd like to be connected with health-care or community support resources.

JOURNEY ON THE TERMINAL TRAIL

"*I now speak openly and honestly about death and dying and encourage the patient and his family to do the same.*"

–Long-term-care nurse, Helenwood, TN

"*I treat my dying patients as if they were members of my own family.*"

–Critical-care nurse, Chicago, IL

"*I compartmentalize my life. Work is work, it stays there; my home life stays at home. It took me a while to figure that one out.*"

–Medical nurse, St. Catharine's, Ontario

"Helping families make the decision about when to withdraw life support was hard at first. Now I believe that sometimes death can be a natural thing."

–Critical-care nurse, Roseville, MI

"Nurses are not able to reverse a patient's grave prognosis, but we can offer the patient compassion, support, understanding, and knowledge."

–Pediatric nurse, El Cerrito, CA

HELPING PATIENTS' FAMILIES FACE DEATH

No matter what health-care setting you work in, it is possible that you may need to assist a bereaved family. Here are some thoughts:

Do:

- **Answer questions from the patient's relatives.** Let them know details about the death if they were not able to be present. The fact that the patient was not in pain, looked peaceful, or died in her sleep might be comforting to them.

- **Make a referral to chaplain or social workers' services, if available.** These professionals have vast experience in dealing with grief and can help connect the family to further sources of support in the community.

- **Let the family know about other sources of support for their grieving process.** Include sites on the Internet that offer support for mourners, such as GriefNet (at *www.griefnet.org*) and Growth House, Inc. (at *www.growthhouse.org*).

Don't:

- **Rush the family members from contact with their loved one;** they might need some private time with him.

- **Make judgments about the response of the family to the actual death.** At such an emotional time, people can say and do things that are not characteristic of their usual behavior.

- **Be afraid** to show your own emotions at the loss.

WORKING WITH THE FAMILY AFTER DEATH

"Be forthright with patients and families in regard to disease process and prognosis. Families really appreciate the honesty."

–Critical-care nurse, Rio Rancho, NM

"I try to stay with the family as much as possible, and when I feel they are ready, I direct them: It's time to go home, it's time to call a funeral home, etc. I have found that it seems to be a relief for them to be told that it's all right to go home and what their next step needs to be."

–Emergency department nurse, Berlin, NJ

"*It's really difficult to stand next to a mother of a 20-year-old who is dying and keep my composure. I found that when I would personalize such a situation (thinking it was my brother . . .), it made it hard to deal with. But setting aside thoughts of my family helped me to help those patients and families deal with their own situations.*"

—Critical-care nurse, Louisville, KY

RECOVERING YOUR SENSE OF HEALING

When a patient's struggle to live is over, you will not only be dealing with his family's emotions, but also with your own feelings of loss and frustration.

Do:

- **Remember that it's okay for you to be upset,** too, even if you've only known the patient a short while.
- **Document the interventions that you made to make the patient comfortable at the end.** It will help you remember that you were there when the patient and family needed you the most.
- **Talk about your feelings to your colleagues and your family.** You don't have to be the "strong, silent type."

Don't:

- **Rehash more than once how you dealt with the patient and what you could do better next time.** Review and move on. You will use the good ideas you came up with next time.
- **Blame yourself for events and situations beyond your sphere of influence;** you can only do so much. Death is not an event that can be controlled.
- **Forget to seek professional assistance yourself,** if you are suffering symptoms of burnout.

HEALING THE HEALER

"*Talk about death with other nurses. They will understand and help you.*"

    –Intensive care unit nurse, Huntington Beach, CA

"*Dealing with death was difficult at first, because I felt like I didn't know what to do. Now I realize that death is something we all must go through.*"

    –Surgical nurse, Mauldin, SC

"*I use the chaplain services of my hospital for myself as well as for my patients. Talking with a minister, priest, or rabbi can really help.*"

    –Intensive care unit nurse, San Antonio, TX

As you read this chapter's caregiving challenges and discovered how experienced nurses conquered them, you must have said to yourself, "How can I cope with that much stress and still take care of patients?" The best answer is, let your coworkers help you. In the next chapter, experienced nurses will share their hard-won insights about how to gain rapport with your new colleagues.

CHAPTER 6

Rapport with Coworkers

"No one can understand a nurse like another nurse."
–Intensive care unit nurse, Columbia, MD

Once you're hired, you'll be so busy with orientation, patient care, and policies and procedures that you won't have a lot of spare time to get to know your coworkers. And when you finally do find some respite, how can you bond with your colleagues? In this chapter, seasoned nurses share tips on becoming—and staying—a fully accepted member of the team.

IMPRESSING YOUR SUPERVISOR

The first person you'll want to get to know on your team is your supervisor. One sure way to impress your supervisor is to give good, solid patient care without being a high-maintenance employee. Here are some tips:

Do:

- **Volunteer for challenging patient-care assignments.** Not only will you stretch your ability, but you will show initiative.

- **Be willing to schedule some personal time to read about your organization and unfamiliar patient-care techniques.** This way, you can ask solid questions and get useful answers to increase your clinical knowledge from the beginning. Put thank-you notes from patients or their families in your personal folder.

- **Keep a list of all your ongoing educational activities,** both in and outside your work setting.

Don't:

- **Underestimate the skills you bring to the job;** think of at least one positive characteristic that adds value (such as enthusiasm, willingness to work hard, or being good with kids).
- **Think that if you make a mistake, your career in health care is over;** you have to learn the right way to proceed, and then move forward.

LOOKING UP TO YOUR LEADER

"*Maintain a friendly relationship with your boss, ask to go to workshops, and set goals every six months to aspire to.*"

   –Medical-surgical nurse, Mt. Pleasant, SC

"*Make sure your work is completed, and not half-done, which leaves the nurse who follows you to finish it.*"

   –Home-care nurse, Center, TX

Prove to them you know what you are doing. Be honest, be credible, and stay out of the politics.

—OB-GYN nurse, Madison, WI

Some supervisors may not seem nice, but they're just trying to make sure you're a safe nurse. Don't appear to take it personally.

—Emergency department nurse, Broken Arrow, OK

Seek every opportunity to perform a new skill, care for a new type of patient, or do anything else that will broaden your scope of experience.

—OB-GYN nurse, Claremont, CA

"Have compassion for your patients, confidence in your training, pride in your career, and the ability to ask for help when you need it."

–Nurse practitioner, Nashville, TN

"Go to work each day with a clean slate and begin again. Be flexible and be a team player."

–Oncology nurse, St. Paul, MN

"I took every continuing education class offered by our education department my first year out of nursing school. That looked impressive on my first evaluation."

–Critical-care nurse, Fayetteville, NC

> "*I showed up to work on time EVERY DAY.*"
>
> **–Hospital staff nurse, Knoxville, TN**

WORKING WITH YOUR TEAMMATES

Establishing a positive professional relationship with your coworkers can be an easy task—if you go into the situation with the right frame of mind. Your approach is critical. Consider the suggestions below:

Do:

- **Communicate honestly.** Your reputation should be that people can count on you for straightforward factual information and for thoughtful opinions.

Don't:

- **Be arrogant, try to fake perfection, or blame others** for your mistakes.

● **Listen to juicy gossip and pass along tidbits you have gathered.** Some workplaces are like a soap opera, but it is prudent to avoid contributing to that distraction.

● **Complain about your workload,** your hours, your equipment, your commute, your everything. . . . Misery might love company, but you don't want to diminish morale.

● **Overlook your fellow newcomers as a source of support.** It can take just one talk with a coworker to make all the difference in your outlook!

STOP, LOOK, AND LISTEN

"*Feel out the unit before opening up too much. Let them get to know you on a professional level before you get too comfortable.*"
   –Intensive care unit nurse, Parkton, MD

"*Observe a lot. Coworkers learn to respect you when they are confident that you understand patient care principles.*"
   –Critical-care nurse, North Highlands, CA

"*Remember: Everyone has something to offer, and people love being asked for advice.*"

–OB-GYN nurse, Baltimore, MD

"*Most times, if you ask for help, other nurses will help you, but if you don't ask, they will watch you flounder.*"

–Medical telemetry nurse, Kunkletown, PA

THE AXE OF ARROGANCE

"*First and foremost, be willing to learn. I have noticed a lot of new nurses coming in with a 'know-it-all' attitude. Your coworkers will not appreciate it, and you will end up knowing less. I accepted the fact that the experienced nurses knew way more than I did.*"

–Pediatric nurse, Chicago, IL

"I have found that more experienced nurses can spot a mile away new nurses who act as though they know everything."

–Intensive care unit nurse, Syracuse, NY

"I admit that I am not perfect. I make mistakes and sometimes I am wrong in the way I see things, so I listen to advice from others. I am just one part of the team."

–Long-term-care nurse, Oak Ridge, TN

DON'T ADD TO THE RUMOR MILL

"Keep your mouth shut about rumors and talking about other nurses. Your seemingly innocent comments might have a way of returning and biting you back."

–Surgical nurse, Farber, MO

"Be kind and friendly to everyone . . . even if you don't like them!"

  –Operating room nurse, Owings Mills, MD

"Don't take sides with coworkers; stay neutral. You never know who is going to make it up the ladder and have power over your future."

  –Pediatric nurse, Ft. Myers, FL

"Camaraderie is essential. Positive people don't talk about each other. I am on the night shift and we are like a little family, because we have to work so closely together to successfully take care of the volume of patients that we have."

  –Orthopedic nurse, Seabrook, TX

THE SOCIAL SCENE

Don't forget that befriending your coworkers has a bonus built in. Not only does it help you work better as a team, but you'll be spending your workday with people you actually want to share your life with! Not sure how to break the ice? Try these suggestions:

Do:

- **Make the effort to get to know your colleagues from the start.** Put the date of your one-month anniversary on your calendar, so that if you have not done much socializing previously, you can surprise your teammates with bagels to celebrate together.

- **Share some of yourself.** Bring in some inexpensive items to share with your coworkers, such as unused coupons, books, or professional journals that you have finished reading. Post an article of interest on the bulletin board. It's the little things that show you care! Invite coworkers to share breaks and meals together with you on a routine basis. Make sure you don't overlook anybody.

- **Accept invitations to group get-togethers or initiate them yourself . . .** even something simple such as going to a movie together.

Don't:

- **Limit yourself to just discussing the workload and patient-care issues.** There is a world of possibilities for what you might have in common.
- **Feel that your relationship is confined to work hours.** Enjoy the company of your coworkers in another (and usually more informal) environment. Meet them for drinks after work. Tour museums or attend concerts together. Plan activities such as holiday parties or shopping trips.

BIRDS OF A FEATHER WORK WELL TOGETHER

"*It helped me to find just one nurse who had similar tastes and work techniques to hang out with.*"

–Surgical nurse, Farber, MO

"Luckily, there were other nurses who were starting at the same time as I was. We all stuck together and made sure we went out together to de-stress."

–Intensive care unit nurse, Columbia, MD

"Form bonds with other new nurses, because they are going through the same thing you are going through."

–OB-GYN nurse, Baltimore, MD

DANCE OF DIALOGUE

"Just take the time to ask them how their day is going."

–Oncology nurse, Orlando, FL

"Learn your coworkers' names quickly and at least one interesting thing about them. Then, make a point to call the person by name and bring the item up in casual conversation. Everyone likes to feel important!"

–Surgical nurse, Winston-Salem, NC

"I asked them about themselves; after a while, they started asking me questions about my life."

–Orthopedic nurse, Seabrook, TX

"Know when they are available for conversation and when they are not because they are too stressed with their patients."

–Critical-care nurse, Hamden, CT

THERE'S NO "I" IN "TEAM"

Your new coworkers have an unwritten rating scale to judge how much of a team player everyone is. If you want to be on the upper part of the scale, make a conscious effort to do the following:

Do:

- **Look around to see if anything needs to be done if you have a few minutes of downtime.** Initiate action, rather than waiting to be asked or told.

- **Be willing to do the little tasks that can fall through the cracks,** like cleaning the staff refrigerator or microwave, organizing the patients' reading materials, or taking down old announcements from bulletin boards. Get to know how to sense your teammates' nonverbal SOSs. You will see from their facial expressions that they look harried, or hear them sigh (not in relief), or realize that they haven't joined you for a meal. Even if they don't ask—pitch in.

Don't:

- **Think of your coworkers on the team as a hierarchy of levels.** Help everyone equally.

- **Take the help of others for granted**—let them know you appreciate it.

SUPPORTING TEAM EFFORTS

"*We are all a team. By ensuring the success of our team, we ensure our own success.*"

   –Critical-care nurse, Norridge, IL

"*Follow up throughout the day—we need to frequently communicate and update each other on how the patients are doing.*"

   –Pediatric nurse, Provo, UT

"*We all work together. Before the day is over, we make sure that all our nurses are caught up and stay if they need help. We don't let each other drown.*"

–Oncology nurse, Orlando, FL

"*We stick by each other, because the job can be very stressful. Even helping a coworker in the most basic way can make your coworker's day much easier.*"

–Hospital staff nurse, Braintree, MA

GETTING ATTUNED TO THE TEAM'S MUSIC

"*No one should be sitting down in the nurses' station unless everyone is.*"

–Emergency room nurse, Santa Clarita, CA

"Help everyone as much as you can without hurting the care of your patients. It's true that what goes around comes around."

–Critical-care nurse, Searcy, AR

"Even if you don't know how to do everything on your unit in the beginning, you can still help out with the basics. Help get vitals, pick up a phone, or answer a call light."

–OB-GYN nurse, St. Louis, MO

"I know I required a lot of help from my coworkers at first, so I made sure to express my appreciation for their knowledge, assistance, and patience and how it impacted my experience as a new nurse."

–Pediatric nurse, El Cerrito, CA

DEALING WITH DIFFICULT COWORKERS

You already know that you can't get along with everyone all of the time. But that doesn't make it any easier when you come across coworkers who are almost impossible to work with. Accept the inevitable and learn how to avoid a negative outcome for yourself and, ultimately, for your patients.

Do:

● **Keep the situation in perspective.** Recognize that conflicts have many causes: from thoughtless remarks, clumsy attempts at being witty, needing to not feel overlooked, or a simple misunderstanding of words, to an honest difference of opinion. Don't automatically assume that the coworker has a problem with you.

● **Ask your mentor or close friend to act as a sounding board before you decide how to handle the conflict.** An outsider can give you practical and objective advice.

Don't:

- **Wait until you can't stand it anymore to deal with multiple instances of disrespect.** Denial of conflict will not make it go away.

- **Send an email, write a quick note, or leave a voice-mail message for the person.** Your words, however well intentioned and well phrased, could be misinterpreted.

- **Get overly emotional when expressing your side of the story.** People won't be able to understand what you are saying while you are crying.

- **Run the other way when faced with conflict.** Instead, try to spend more personal time with that person. Chances are, you'll find you have more in common than you thought.

- **Worry that you will have to endure the difficult situation forever.** People switch jobs, individuals change, and over time, it might be you who alters your perception or response.

RULES OF THE ROAD

"Be open-minded about others' views and nursing styles."

—OB-GYN nurse, Columbus, OH

"*Coworkers may not always accept you at first; some may never accept you. Know who are your 'reference' people to go to and who to stay far away from.*"

   –Emergency department nurse, Egg Harbor Township, NJ

"*I worked with one nurse who was notorious for not being a team player. I consistently asked her what I could do for her and helped her when she needed it. One day I was really busy and went to get a room ready for a patient, and the other nurse had already done it for me.*"

   –OB-GYN nurse, Claremont, CA

"*You can't work as a team if there is tension. We have to help resolve issues between our teammates when they are stressed. This will be better for everyone in the long run.*"

   –Neurology nurse, Albuquerque, NM

HAVING A POSITIVE ATTITUDE

You enjoy working with others who look at the bright side of a situation. Similarly, if you approach your own tasks with a sense of optimism and enthusiasm, it's bound to rub off on other people!

Do:

- **Keep alert for the good things that happen** so you can be grateful for them as they occur. Share them with your coworkers.
- **Listen to your language:** Is it full of words expressing negativity ("We are never going to get this done")? A negative outlook, even when unintentional, can bring the team down.

Don't:

- **Take things personally.** Whether nature provided you with a "thin skin" or a "thick skin" as your response to criticism, don't let others' opinions get in the way of your continual improvement.
- **Be your own worst enemy;** don't get down on yourself. Instead, think of yourself as your best cheerleader. Rah! Rah!

STAY UPBEAT

"*Memorize 'Hey, let me know if you need anything.' When nurses know they have support, they can perform at their best.*"

–Emergency room nurse, Kansas City, MO

"*A happy disposition will get you more miles ahead with your coworkers than being negative. Be even nicer to the ones who aren't receptive to you. Kill 'em with kindness!*"

–OB-GYN nurse, Fort Riley, KS

"*Every Friday we have 'Feel the Love Friday.' Each week is a different theme. We then bring in different foods according to that theme, such as football Friday, pasta Friday, junk food Friday.*"

–Medical telemetry nurse, Brick, NJ

"If you don't have a sense of humor, get one."

–Emergency room nurse, Rancho Santa Fe, CA

I love to laugh, and so I sometimes will come to work and tell a funny story that happened to me during my time off work. That story usually sets a lighter tone for the floor, as other coworkers who might usually be negative will also share a humorous tale.

–Orthopedic nurse, Seabrook, TX

Instead of starting as a member of the team, what if you are immediately put in the position of leading the team? Can you quickly combine your current clinical knowledge and potential leadership skills to direct the work of others effectively? Don't spend time wondering—the next chapter will tell you just how to do that!

CHAPTER 7

Leading the Troops

"Keep it democratic—don't play favorites."
—Emergency department nurse, Kansas City, MO

One of the most exciting and scary aspects of being a new nurse is that your first assignment might be to lead a patient-care team. Often your team members have been working together (without your leadership) for some time. They have considerable experience and strong opinions about getting the job done. Now you must step into the situation and take charge. How do you successfully delegate with ease and confidence? By reading the input of nurses who discovered the secrets of team-tested team-leading techniques!

APPROACHING THE TASK OF DELEGATING

The main responsibility you have as team leader is assigning tasks to your people. The trick is to delegate the workload so that patients receive timely care, while keeping team morale up by not overloading any member of your staff. Sometimes, you will find it hard to achieve a balance, but these tips should keep you on track:

- **Give everyone, including yourself, a second (and third) chance** to prove their merit.
- **Don't be quick to judge** any member of your team. The slowest person might be the most careful; the most talkative might energize the patients.
- **Be clear** about what needs to be accomplished, and be open to answering questions and responding to comments at the start and the end of the workday.
- **Gather data** about how well particular assignments have been accomplished.
- **Be receptive** to feedback from your team.

● **Adjust your recipe as necessary;** experimenting is part of the learning process.

KEY CONCEPTS TO SUCCESSFUL DELEGATING

"*A nurse is on the front lines. You have the opportunity to be everything for a patient from informing the patient of the doctor's plans to making a peanut butter sandwich; however, it is important to delegate such non-RN tasks to those more appropriate for the task.*"

–Medical-surgical nurse, St. Paul, MN

"*Treat everyone with equal respect; we're all people. It's always good to ask rather than to demand, and to keep in mind that we're all here to work together in helping the patients.*"

–Intensive care unit nurse, Columbia, MD

I worked a lot of overtime until I learned to say, 'I'm not able to help you right now,' to the nurse's aides I work with. This was incredibly difficult because I truly wanted to be an active part of the team, not just the team leader. And if I was signing my name to something, I wanted to ensure it was done well. However, learning to delegate well was vital. There is definitely not enough time for me to do it all.

–Long-term-care nurse, Gaston, OR

I discuss patient care with the nursing assistant at the beginning of the shift to avoid any misunderstandings. I encourage communication between myself and the nursing assistants. I thank them for their help at the end of the shift.

–Hospital staff nurse, Whispering Pines, NC

" *As I am getting report, I put sticky notes on the pull-down outside of each patient's room. After report, I find each of my aides and verbally tell them I left notes and what each note says for each patient. That way, they can't use the excuse that I didn't tell them about what they are supposed to accomplish before the end of the shift.* "

–Orthopedic nurse, Seabrook, TX

MATCHING STAFF WITH ASSIGNMENTS

Here's how to best match your team's workload and your nursing staff's skills:

" *Delegation largely depends on how well you know the capabilities of each member of your staff as compared to the patients' cases and demand for care. Also consider the ratio of patients to staff and the proximity of the patients, so that your team doesn't end up running from one end of the unit to the other.* "

–Psychiatric nurse, Elmendorf, TX

"*I try to keep assignments fair and equal. Each person has strengths and likes and weaknesses and dislikes that come into play. I try to assign a mix so each person has some tasks they enjoy doing and a few they don't.*"

–Long-term-care nurse, Oak Ridge, TN

"*I assign patients to nurses who I know will be able to handle them and are comfortable with them.*"

–Psychiatric nurse, San Diego, CA

COMMUNICATING ASSIGNMENTS

"*Don't play 'See you later, delegator.' Once you assign duties, you need to be clear about your expectations and make sure to follow up! Write the assignments down. I find that directives are harder to ignore if they are in writing.*"

–Rehabilitation nurse, Winter Park, FL

"*Be clear and thorough, ask if there are questions, and state your expectations.*"

–Dermatology nurse, Chicago, IL

"*I always ask if they are familiar with the task, tell them to report back to me, and if they're unsure about something, not to hesitate to ask for clarification.*"

–Pediatric nurse, Ocala, FL

"*Don't forget 'please' and 'thank you.' Always follow up.*"

–Intensive care unit nurse, Parkton, MD

"*Sometimes it will be necessary to compromise; don't take it as a sign of failure.*"

–Rehabilitation nurse, Barnesville, GA

"*Give clear, precise, understandable steps to accomplish the task and always check back with them for the results or offer help if needed. Delegate kindly; no one likes to be bossed around.*"

–Operating room nurse, San Antonio, TX

"*I try not to be short with the help that I receive. A nursing assistant can make a day so much better, and they are working just as hard as you. At the beginning of the day, I try to talk to them to see how their workload is, and figure out how we can get everything done that our patients need.*"

–Hospital staff nurse, Chicago, IL

TRAINING STAFF

Some jobs will even ask you to train your team within weeks of your arrival. How are you supposed to train people when you're newer at the job than they are? Don't worry—your schooling provided you with the basic tools you need to succeed, and this book will do the rest! Here are some guidelines:

Do:

- **Practice in front of a sympathetic colleague or mentor** at least once so that you feel confident in your presentation. If no one is available, record your rehearsal or present it in front of a mirror, and evaluate yourself.
- **Recognize that not everyone on your team has had the benefit of the same background.** Your job is not to equalize the past, but to focus on the critical clinical skills or procedures needed in the present.
- **Show the technique.** If you don't want to illustrate the procedure on an actual patient, ask for a volunteer staff person or use a dummy or an anatomical model of an organ.
- **Keep it simple.** Your audience is less likely to absorb long-winded lessons than brief, specific action points.

Don't:

- **Avoid questions** from your staff about the impact on their workloads of trying new methods.

- **Feel you have to perform a complete educational transfusion in one sitting;** sometimes it takes time for the full content to sink in.
- **Forget to use handouts as you speak.** Post them on the staff bulletin board after your training so staff not able to attend can gain some idea of what they missed.

SOME TEACHING TIPS

"*I teach how it is to be done, I show how to do it, I help them do it, I watch them do it, and then I let go.*"

–Critical-care nurse, Virginia Beach, VA

"*Get to know your staff and recognize who needs to be constantly supervised.*"

–Medical telemetry nurse, Pico Rivera, CA

"You need to be very familiar with equipment and procedures, and you need to be organized. Otherwise the staff will question your competency."

–Critical-care nurse, North Highlands, CA

PARTICIPATE IN THE WORKLOAD YOURSELF

During the delegation process, remember to assign some tasks to yourself. Experienced nurses reported this as the single most effective technique to motivate the entire team. Here's their nuts-and-bolts approach:

Do:

● **Recognize that the schedule of patient-care needs might have a roller-coaster pattern;** you need to pitch in full-time today, but that does not mean that you will be so totally involved tomorrow.

Don't:

- **Rescue people from bad judgments they made about pacing themselves;** assist them rather than taking over.

- **Forget that your participation in hands-on care is keeping your clinical skills fresh.** You don't want to get rusty.

- **Hesitate to ask for instructions in accomplishing a task from any member of your team,** whether that team member is licensed or unlicensed. This shows the democratic nature of your leadership.

CHARGING THE TEAM'S BATTERIES

"I feel that staff nurses and technicians have more respect for a charge nurse or manager who is not afraid of direct patient care or working hard."

–Emergency room nurse, New York, NY

" *I began working as a charge nurse and preceptor to new staff in my first six months as an RN, which was a real challenge. It is important to never ask someone to do something that you would not do yourself. Even though you're in charge, you have to establish yourself as a team player.* "

–Medical-surgical nurse, Mt. Pleasant, SC

" *I wouldn't ask a nurse tech to make a bed if I wasn't busy myself. But I would ask them if I needed to pass meds, because that is something the nurse tech can't do.* "

–Medical-surgical nurse, Kansas City, MO

A SUPPORTIVE ENVIRONMENT

You spend a significant amount of your life at work. You want to be in a welcoming environment—and your coworkers will agree heartily. If you're the team leader, it's a given that other people are supposed to follow your directions. Within this structure, does it feel to them like a rigid hierarchy? Do they feel micromanaged? Or ignored? From the start, you want to create a culture that values teamwork. You can do this by:

- Listening to the members of your team when they seem to be complaining. Is it possible that their assignments actually are overwhelming?

- Letting people save face when their mistakes are discussed. Assume their goodwill and competence—allow them ample opportunity to make changes.

- Giving compliments. Let the members of your team know how their contribution is important and how the outcome of their work made a difference to patients, families, and colleagues. When people take pride in their work, they work even harder!

THE POWER OF POSITIVITY

"*Be a mentor rather than a boss.*"

   –Urology nurse, Kalamazoo, MI

"*Tell them you really appreciate what they are doing. Encourage them.*"

   –Pediatric nurse, Provo, UT

"*Delegate very delicately. I always try to be fair, and even though it gets tiring, I give explanations for my reasoning. I also listen to them and offer any help I can.*"

   –Telemetry nurse, Dubois, PA

"*Know that you will not please everyone. Treat each employee individually—each deals with stress differently.*"

   –Nurse educator, House Springs, MO

"Be friends with those you supervise, but keep it a professional relationship. That way they will not take orders too personally."

–Oncology nurse, Beggs, OK

Now that you have heard about successful methods of contributing to your team's cohesiveness and delegating work assignments to your staff, you are in a good position to learn how to effectively work with physicians and other clinicians. In the next chapter, experienced nurses will tell you how to build a positive and productive relationship with them.

CHAPTER 8

Helping Doctors Help Patients

"The relationship between nurses and doctors comes down to respecting each other's roles and working together for the good of the patients."

–Ambulatory-care nurse, Baltimore, MD

Healing is a complex process that calls for the cohesive partnering of efforts between patients, nurses, and doctors. Earlier in this book, you learned solid methods of establishing rapport with patients and with coworkers. Now you can complete the triangle of care by discovering this chapter's secrets to building strong, positive relationships with physicians.

Sometimes doctors and nurses look at clinical and administrative issues from different angles, and this can cause conflicts. This chapter will help you cope with those situations as well. So read on to find out how to make your contact with doctors a consistent win-win situation for patient care.

GAINING DOCTORS' RESPECT

The surest way to build a positive relationship with physicians is to gain their respect. Your first step is to recognize that your roles are intertwined—and that you are in charge of what you contribute to the dialogue and your response to how the situation unfolds. Here are some tips for building a strong foundation for rapport:

Do:

- **Introduce yourself with your full name,** as the nurse for a particular patient or group of patients.
- **Give doctors a concise picture of their patient's status.** Let them know what worked well and what didn't. State your assessment of what further care is needed.
- **Share compliments from patients and their family members** about the work of the entire care team.

Don't:

- **Rush through giving details about patients.** If time is critical, prioritize relaying only the information needing immediate response.
- **End your discussion without clearly understanding the follow-up plan** (i.e., when does the doctor next want you to contact her with details about changes in the patient's condition?).
- **Agree to take on tasks that you cannot successfully accomplish.** If you are short-staffed, say so. If a piece of equipment is unavailable, explain the alternatives. If there is a waiting list, communicate that fact.

PROFESSIONAL AND COLLEGIAL

"*It was helpful to tell the docs that I just started. That let them know I was new, not incompetent.*"

–Emergency room nurse, Osage, IA

"*Become friendly with all of the doctors. Talk to them, learn from them, show interest. The more the doctors get to know you, the easier it gets!*"

–Intensive care unit nurse, Virginia Beach, VA

"*Interact with accuracy, professionalism, and politeness.*"

–Pediatric nurse, Bedford, NY

All doctors' personalities are different. Some doctors expect more than others. Some are laid back. Others will yell at every little thing. I have learned to cope by recognizing that doctors have bad days just as we do.

–OB-GYN nurse, Kansas City, MO

Get a second opinion about a situation the doctor and you disagree about, just to make sure that you're seeing things in the right light and not missing something.

–Intensive care unit nurse, Lynchburg, VA

Doctors don't have tolerance for new nurses if they show immaturity, lack interest, or pretend that they know what they are doing when they don't. Honesty, integrity, and willingness to listen and be helpful are universal positive traits.

–Urology nurse, Kalamazoo, MI

"Older doctors can really intimidate a new nurse by asking questions the nurse doesn't know the answers to in front of the patient. But in the long run, they're helping. That happened to me, and I went home and learned all I could about that subject so the next time I would know the answers."

–Surgical nurse, Farber, MO

"Doctors may not have been introduced to the role of nursing in their schooling. I help them understand our role by being active in discussing patient issues and understanding rationales for why certain medications or treatments or plans are used."

–Ambulatory-care nurse, Baltimore, MD

SURVEY SAYS: BE ASSERTIVE

"*When the physicians expect X number of things to be done in too short a time period, just tell them how it is. That there is only one of you.*"

–Critical-care nurse, Hamden, CT

"*I used to get offended if physicians were short with me. Now I just keep in mind that most people are stressed and do not let myself be intimidated. If I became intimidated by another health-care professional and did not voice my opinion, I would be compromising the patient's care.*"

–Orthopedic nurse, Philadelphia, PA

"Some physicians will try to push you around. If you show them that you have confidence, they are less likely to do this. Never let anyone speak to you in an abusive manner. This should be reported to your supervisor for immediate action."

–OB-GYN nurse, St. Louis, MO

"I was pushed by anesthesia and surgeons to hurry through checking in the patient and getting the room ready for surgery. Now I tell them that we are not taking the patient into the room until I check everything. I don't let them rush me. All these steps are necessary for the safety of the patient."

–Operating room nurse, St. Catharine's, Ontario

"I work nights. It is difficult knowing when to call the doctor and what questions can wait until morning. Asking your coworkers' opinions is really helpful."

–Critical-care nurse, Topeka, KS

SMOOTHING ROUGH WATERS

If there is some difference of opinion or perceived lack of collegiality, experienced nurses suggest various approaches:

"If a doctor or other member of the team is being disrespectful or rude, they need to be told privately. Chances are, they didn't realize how they were acting."

–Intensive care unit nurse, Columbia, MD

"If I feel tension between myself and the physician, I make sure before the end of the day to ask personally what is wrong. My openness really helps, because at times doctors will not make the first move."

–Allergy clinic nurse, Gardena, CA

"I am direct and ask the physician or other clinician what I should have noticed or done differently in the given situation."

—Emergency room nurse, Rancho Santa Fe, CA

DISCUSSING PATIENT-CARE ISSUES

While final patient-care decisions are ultimately up to doctors, many of their decisions are based on information you provide and suggestions you offer. Want to make sure you are heard when you have an idea or opinion? Try the following approach:

- Remember that you are on the same team, not on opposing sides. Don't be hostile or automatically expect a rejection of your input.

- Appreciate that the physician is trying to get work done in a time-limited situation.

- If you can anticipate what is needed for decision-making (charts, lab results, vital signs), pull those facts together to present as a package.

- If you made notes on patient-care issues needing physician input, comfortably refer to them, checking them off once completed. Then you won't miss something and need to contact the doctor later.

- If you can't come to an agreement about a treatment for the patient, you need to get a more experienced staff person involved in a professional manner. Patient safety is the goal; never forget that.

TALKING TO DOCTORS

"For the most part, physicians want just the facts. They don't need to hear a whole spiel on the patient."

–Renal unit nurse, Leawood, KS

"Physicians will ask you why you did something, and they expect you to know the rationale behind it. Explain your decision-making process."

–OB-GYN nurse, Fort Riley, KS

"Speaking up to physicians about a patient's care was hard to do at first. There was this invisible wall I had put between the doctors and myself. I was only a nurse and they were the doctors. I came to realize that I am the one who is there with the patient constantly, and I need to be an active part of the plan of care— the patient's well-being is at risk."

–OB-GYN nurse, St. Louis, MO

"I learned to take a deep breath and think before I spoke."
–Cardiology nurse, Mamaroneck, NY

QUESTIONING THE DOCTOR

Now that you feel comfortable having basic conversations with physicians, let's up the ante. How about when you have to confront them with news that differs from what they expected or disagree with their plan of care or don't want to carry out orders that you feel will endanger the patient? Here's a solid approach:

- Be objective. Limit yourself to the facts of the matter, without passing judgment on why it happened.

- Broach your point in the form of a question, "Do you think that the patient would benefit from . . . ?" instead of harshly criticizing the current care plan.

- Review your concerns ahead of time with a seasoned coworker to see if you need further research or patient-care data to support your opinion.

THE HARD-TO-HAVE DISCUSSIONS

"*Speak up. Question their actions if you feel they need to be questioned. Do not delay your concerns.*"

   –Emergency room nurse, Hagerstown, MD

"*I ask myself, How important is this conflict? Is it life-threatening to the patient? Will anyone be hurt by this situation?*"

   –Critical-care nurse, Roseville, MI

"Always go with your gut feeling. I was forced to confront a physician with inappropriate medication orders, and much to my surprise, he was very appreciative."

–Orthopedic nurse, Winona, MN

"As a new nurse, I was not always sure of routines and standards of practice in the community for my patient population. If I questioned a physician and he in turn questioned me, I would back down. Now I am sure of routines and standards of practice, so I can stand my ground."

–OB-GYN nurse, Claremont, CA

DIALING THE DOCTOR

You are going to have to contact the patients' physicians by pager or telephone at all hours of the day and possibly the night. The timing and the need to condense your words into a concise report present challenges.

The best approach is to be well prepared:

- Collect all the patient-care information in front of you before you initiate the contact.
- Write the information you receive directly into the clinical record, so you make fewer transcription errors.
- Have an extra pen in case the first one runs out in the middle of your note-taking.
- Call from the quietest area in your workplace.
- If you can't hear or don't understand, ask again.
- If a crucial question occurs to you shortly after you hang up, take a deep breath, mentally confirm that you need the answer, and call again. (Red faces are never seen over the phone!)

PHONING THE PHYSICIAN

"*Unless it is an emergency, call the doctor once with multiple issues rather than calling for little things throughout the day.*"

–Oncology nurse, Orlando, FL

"Evaluate the situation before you call the physician. Can it wait until they make rounds?"

–Hospital staff nurse, Hampton, VA

"Calling physicians while working nights is always tough. It helps to remember that they get paid to do their job . . . just like I do. I always keep a positive attitude on the phone, which makes it harder for a doctor to get too upset."

–Intensive care unit nurse, Franklin, OH

"I have discovered that there are times when you just have to keep calling the doctor to let him know that a patient needs whatever he needs. So if it takes five phone calls before the doctor responds and takes you seriously, then it's worth it."

–Medical-surgical nurse, Lynchburg, VA

" *When you need to contact a physician after rounds, sometimes you have to call the office or service several times before you get a response. I learned that if it is imperative that I speak to her, I demand that I get a call back. I also remind the office or service of how many times I have tried to contact her.* "

–Rehabilitation nurse, Bridgeport, NJ

RELATING TO RESIDENTS

If you are employed in a teaching hospital, you will be working alongside medical students, interns, and residents. They have the same dual responsibility that you had on a clinical rotation—delivering patient care in an on-the-job classroom—and are under a lot of pressure. Here's what nurses ask that you remember when working with them:

"We have many interns and residents who aren't very experienced. I have walked a new doctor through many unfamiliar bedside procedures. They remember that kind of thing and respect me for it."

–Telemetry nurse, Townsend, DE

"I let the residents know about our clinical protocols and what needs to be done. Normally (if it's a new resident) they will listen and give me the appropriate verbal order."

–Cardiology nurse, Morristown, NJ

"When I disagree with a resident's orders, I just ask the resident about it directly; I find that he likes to discuss options with you rather than deciding on his own."

–Critical-care nurse, Newtown, PA

IT'S ALL ABOUT THE PATIENTS

"*In the end, your goal matches the motivation of physicians— the best patient care given in a timely and effective manner. I remind clinicians that the nurses are their eyes and ears when they are not present.*"

   –Home-care nurse, Center, TX

"*Always stand your ground for your patient's safety. Without nurses, the physicians and other clinicians would not be able to provide care to the patients.*"

   –Oncology nurse, Georgetown, KY

"*Always do what you think is right and keep the patient's safety and health in mind. If you do that, you will find that you are working together with the doctor. We are all 'practicing medicine' together.*"

   –Critical-care nurse, Norridge, IL

Knowing how to build good relationships with physicians will come in handy during your entire nursing career. Another source of inspiration can come from discovering and working with your own personal mentor. How do you find—and make the most of—that special individual who can help you adjust to the realities, positive and negative, of the nursing profession? The next chapter gives a full account of the matter.

CHAPTER 9

The Magic of Mentors

"A mentor is an earthbound guardian angel."
–Ambulatory-care nurse, Palo Alto, CA

With origins in Greek mythology, the word *mentor* means experienced and trusted adviser, friend, and counselor. Your mentor can help you develop your professional skills, knowledge, and insight.

A mentor can make all the difference to your successful introduction to the nursing world. Usually your mentor is not the same person as your already-designated preceptor, who is hired to teach you the ropes, but can be. More likely, you will have to find your own volunteer mentor.

In this chapter, experienced nurses offer insights about the role of this unique and special person in your life.

REASONS TO HAVE A MENTOR

You made it through school without a mentor. You got a job without a mentor. Your new job already brings on a whole new set of people—supervisors, colleagues, trainers, preceptors, fellow commuters. So why should you consider inviting another person into your personal and professional life? Because a mentor serves as your very own advocate—someone who is always there to help you deal with your new surroundings as well as:

- Broaden your perspective on the scope of what you can accomplish in nursing.
- Build your confidence and your knowledge of resources.
- Help you understand the nuances of complex organizational relationships.

- Analyze your mistakes and help you learn from them.
- Give you tips on how to do your job faster and more effectively.
- Unlock the doors to advancement opportunities.
- Act as a positive clinical and/or career role model for you.
- Even out the "bumps" of your career path. And what nurse wouldn't want to have a relationship with someone like that!

MENTORS' REPORT CARD: A+

"*Mentors share from their hearts all they have learned from their mistakes. These are experiences that you can't find in a textbook.*"

–Long-term-care nurse, Martinez, CA

"*Mentors are willing to help you in times of need, stick up for you, give you suggestions, and be someone you can look up to.*"

–Orthopedic nurse, Waterford Works, NJ

"*Mentors are nice and empathetic. They encourage you and praise you for your good work.*"

–Hospital staff nurse, Braintree, MA

CARING MENTORS

"*Without fear, you can ask your mentor questions, express frustrations, or tell her about something new that you did for the first time.*"

–Orthopedic nurse, Gainesville, FL

"*Mentors will let you try new things and not only tell you what they are doing but why they are doing it. They will teach you the little things, such as what parts of the chart to address and how they organize their work.*"

–Hospital staff nurse, Claremont, CA

" *Mentors will let you observe how they function at work. They will show you the 'tricks of the trade.' Use their key insights as a guide for developing your own standards.* "

–OB-GYN nurse, Baltimore, MD

LOCATING YOUR MENTOR

In some working situations, you'll be assigned a mentor. But more often than not, you're on your own. How do you know where to look, or how you should even begin to go about finding a mentor? Here are some tips:

- **Introduce yourself as a new employee to everyone you meet** in formal and informal groups in the workplace: committee meetings, workshops, even the hospital cafeteria. You might find that you click with someone who has similar clinical or professional interests.

- **Check out online resources,** such as *www.nursingcenter.com*, which has a nursing community link called Mentor Connection, or *https:// groups.yahoo.com/neo/groups/PHCC-Nightingales/info*, a website that helps cultivate mentoring relationships between nurses.

- **Look for announcements of local meetings** of nursing specialty groups, and attend the next event they sponsor.
- **Go back to your nursing school and ask your favorite teacher to give you suggestions for mentors.** Or go to a continuing education class and ask the instructor for possible matches.

ON THE TRAIL

" Ask supervisors and charge nurses if they can recommend someone."

–Surgical nurse, Belmont, CA

" I visited the ward prior to starting work and chatted with different people. Don't be afraid to ask who enjoys being a mentor. Usually people will be upfront and honest and let you know who in the workplace would make the best mentors."

–Medical-surgical nurse, Summerville, SC

"My mentor happened to be my preceptor, but it may not always work out that way. An instructor from your nursing school is a possibility. In addition, you may find a new colleague who might take you under his wing."

–Perioperative nurse, El Cerrito, CA

YOUR TIMETABLE

How soon should you choose a mentor? Is it best to jump into that relationship as soon as you get settled on the job? Or should it be a more thoughtful process, where you explore your options? Experienced nurses debated the issue and came up with these recommendations:

"Finding a mentor as quickly as possible will allow you a smoother transition into the new job."

–Surgical nurse, Winston-Salem, NC

"You don't have to spend a long time searching. You want help early in your career. Ask to just observe on your unit for a couple of days. You can identify the natural teachers, the ones who welcome questions. Other nurses easily approach them with questions or problems."

–Orthopedic nurse, Winona, MN

"It is best to wait a year before deciding on a mentor. By that time, you will have a feel for how one acts and you can tell whether she will be a good match with your personality."

–Pediatric nurse, Fort Myers, FL

"Good mentors are hard to find. In your first year, just introduce yourself to as many people as possible. There are so many incredible nurses out there doing a great job. Just keep meeting them and you will find someone whose goals match yours."

–Hospital staff nurse, Baltimore, MD

"When you first start, you might not be aware of the politics of the place. So tread cautiously and just observe, until you know who is on which side. Hopefully, your mentor will be neutral!"

–Ambulatory-care nurse, Palo Alto, CA

QUALITIES OF A QUALITY MENTOR

So you know the basics: how and when to find a mentor. But what should you be looking for in a good mentor? Typically, quality mentors have the following characteristics. A good mentor is:

- A positive role model, a good listener and motivator.
- Discreet and has the best interests of the individual and the organization in mind. That means you can trust that the feelings and information you share will not leave the room in which you shared them.

- Capable of viewing the role of a mentor as a development opportunity for both of you. The best mentors recognize that you are both in a win-win situation.
- Able to give and receive constructive feedback.
- Able to display empathy and understanding.

How are you supposed to know that someone fits the bill ahead of time? There are no guarantees, but nurses use the same skills that they use to assess patients—combining careful observation with some gentle, probing questions. Nurses successful in locating mentors give their advice on the following pages.

CHOOSING A GREAT MENTOR

"1) Find someone who wants to mentor. 2) Find someone who likes nursing. 3) Find someone who has been at that agency for a while and knows the routine of that setting. 4) Find someone whom patients seem to speak highly of, or whom coworkers speak highly of."

–Cardiology nurse, Ellicott City, MD

"*Choose someone who is good at what she does, but who won't eat you alive if you make a mistake.*"

   –Operating room nurse, Gilliam, MO

"*Find a nurturer, someone who will be supportive. This is not necessarily the best nurse on the unit.*"

   –Intensive care unit nurse, San Diego, CA

"*Make sure you see a little of yourself in that person.*"

   –OB-GYN nurse, Jenkintown, PA

BEST MENTOR IS SOMEONE WHO . . .

"*Takes joy in teaching. Look for one who will not belittle you, but who will lift you up.*"

   –Case management nurse, Knoxville, TN

"*You can talk to whenever needed, but when he speaks to you his lingo is not above your level of expertise.*"

–Pediatric nurse, Ocala, FL

"*Is experienced, grounded, and comfortable in her position. Someone who doesn't mind answering questions and helping a new nurse through those first difficult times. Not everyone is cut out for this, but you're really just looking for someone who has a heart.*"

–Hospital staff nurse, Whispering Pines, NC

"*You can get along with, who challenges you and shows confidence in your growing abilities, and then is able to let you 'fly' solo.*"

–Operating room nurse, Barnesville, GA

LOOK FOR A SPECIAL NURSE WHO . . .

"*Is tough, who will grill you about all aspects of the job. It may be a rough ride, but you will come out of it a winner.*"

–**Emergency room nurse, Berlin, NJ**

"*Goes by the book, even if that is not the kind of person you are. It is key to learn the ideal way of doing things first, then find your own style.*"

Emergency room nurse, Santa Clarita, CA

"*You think you could never be as good as. That way you will always be trying harder to be like that person. To this day I know I have to keep trying because now my mentor is a legend in my mind and heart.*"

–**Critical-care nurse, Searcy, AR**

Q AND A: HOW MUCH EXPERIENCE?

Probably no other mentoring issue is more enthusiastically discussed than how long a person should work as a nurse before he is "experienced" enough to mentor. On the next few pages, nurses weigh in with their opinions, but first, here are some questions (and answers) to help you narrow down your choices:

Q: Do I want to know more about this particular organization and how it runs?

A: A more experienced nurse can sometimes fill you in on the historical perspective.

Q: Do I want to have a sounding board free of longstanding agendas?

A: A newer nurse will approach the situation with a fresh eye.

Q: Do I want to focus on a nursing specialty?

A: If so, certifications and advanced courses might make a difference—and either a more or less experienced nurse with that background would be able to give you that guidance.

Q: Do I want to follow in the footsteps of someone who is just one pace ahead of me? Or do I want to be able to hear about the range of approaches that resulted in someone achieving the peak of a successful career?

A: Let's listen to seasoned nurses' opinions of the pros and cons. . . .

VOTES FOR SENIOR NURSES

"*Go for the nurse who teaches in a nursing school. She will know how to educate you and share her resources. If this is not an option, go for the nurse with the most experience. She'll have her own network to share with you.*"

–Hospital staff nurse, Gwynn Oak, MD

"The best advice is to find an older nurse, particularly someone who is influential, to be your mentor and adviser. He can not only help you get on the fast track, but also help you move forward on it!"

–Emergency department nurse, Pickerington, OH

"Find someone who has had several years of experience. That way you get the benefit of her having been there, done that."

–Hospital staff nurse, Milwaukee, WI

VOTES FOR NEWER NURSES

"A mentor is not always the oldest nurse or the nurse who has worked there the longest—sometimes those nurses have old bad habits."

–Ambulatory-care nurse, Rochester, NY

"For me, it was easy. I connect best with those closer to my age and those who have a similar sense of humor . . . it makes it easier to listen to and learn from those people."

   –Critical-care nurse, Louisville, KY

"Look for someone who is not 'burned out.' Some older nurses who have been in nursing forever seem to have the 'Thank God I am retiring soon' attitude."

   –OB-GYN nurse, Chesapeake, VA

HOW TO INVITE SOMEONE TO MENTOR YOU

"Remember to sound positive, not desperate. You aren't going to need all of the person's time—less than an hour per week."

   –Surgical nurse, Winston-Salem, NC

"Be ready to define your idea of a mentor and what you hope to gain from your time together."

—Geriatric nurse, Gaston, OR

"Let her know that you admire her, and are interested in growing professionally. She will probably be honored that you're asking for her assistance."

—Telemetry nurse, Kunkletown, PA

THE INITIAL MEETING WITH YOUR MENTOR

Once you've chosen the right mentor, you have to focus on making the most of your time together. To start out on the right foot when you first meet with your mentor, you should set up:

● The frequency, place, and time for subsequent meetings.

- How other staff (including your supervisor) will be involved without compromising confidentiality.
- Ways in which your mentor can help you. Do you need help with some immediate skill development or assistance with planning your long-range career? Or both? Share your vision of what you would like to have happen, knowing that it could change in the future.
- The agenda of subsequent meetings.
- How you can contact your mentor between organized meetings if need be.

WARNING SIGNALS

"*As wonderful as having a mentor can be, you should be aware of the possibility of a bad match. It's more likely to happen if you are assigned a mentor, but it can occur even when you have explored thoroughly and chosen thoughtfully. Nurses wanted to let you know what to avoid.... First impressions do count for something. If you have a bad feeling on the match from day one, voice it.*"

–Infertility clinic nurse, Mt. Prospect, IL

"*Don't choose someone who just uses you for free labor. You have the rest of your life to work on your own . . . and get paid for it!*"

–Nurse practitioner, Nashville, TN

"*Some nurses are great nurses but bad teachers.*"

–Medical-surgical nurse, Mt. Pleasant, SC

"*Some nurses just go, go, go, and never show you or explain what they're doing.*"

–Emergency room nurse, Broken Arrow, OK

"*If your personalities don't match, it can be a long road!*"

–OB-GYN nurse, Kansas City, MO

" Mentors are great—but everyone is different in the way they do things. Your personality becomes your practice. I like to do things my way in my time, so it can get frustrating to work with someone who does it another way. Just remember to make your practice your own."

–Critical-care nurse, Scranton, PA

FOLLOW-UP MEETINGS

Make sure to not drop the ball once you've started your relationship with your mentor. At your subsequent meetings, be sure to discuss the following topics:

- Your progress since the last meeting.
- Your work-related problems. Your mentor can be a sounding board, encouraging you to identify the pros and cons of your situation and brainstorming some possible courses of action.

- Your training needs. You can give permission for these to be discussed with your supervisor, or you may want to ask your mentor for advice on where she thinks you need additional instruction.

Here are some specific topics of a more personal nature that your mentor might be able to shed some light on:

- The real organizational chart structure and power relationships (sometimes very different from the official ones).
- How to handle particularly difficult individuals or situations.
- How to deal with unsettling turns of events, such as a less-than-enthusiastic performance evaluation or being overlooked for promotion.
- Your successes—and how you can celebrate them together!

BEST PRACTICES OF MENTEES

"*Be really honest with your mentor. When you need to, say, 'Slow down—I don't understand this,' and have your mentor explain the material to you again.*"

–Emergency room nurse, Santa Clarita, CA

"*Take the risk: You must establish a good rapport with the person and be able to trust her with your heart and soul.*"

–Intensive care unit nurse, Syracuse, NY

"*Ask your mentor to be upfront and honest about your skills. Every time you work together, ask him to evaluate your progress. Keep notes on what you need to work on.*"

–Operating room nurse, St. Catharine's, Ontario

IF YOU CAN'T FIND A FORMAL MENTOR

You've searched high. You've searched low. You've searched everywhere! But you can't find a good mentor. What can you do? Three types of individuals make excellent substitutes. Make sure you know how to contact these internal resources:

- **Training and development staff.** These people can direct you to less well known educational resources such as workshops, courses, and library materials. They'll also point out higher education funding opportunities both within and outside your organization.

- **Quality improvement staff.** These people are interested in seeing that all employees are involved in projects to improve the quality and safety of patient care and satisfaction.

- **Nurse recruiter.** If you're looking to move forward in your profession, this person will not only know about other openings before they are posted and the unwritten criteria for hiring specific positions, but also be able to assess your chances of getting a particular job before you even apply.

BROADENING YOUR BASE OF SUPPORT

"As you work on your unit, you will find that you make bonds with many more experienced nurses, and that they can act as resources when you are in need."

–Pediatric nurse, Chicago, IL

" *Pick two to three nurses whom you respect and ask them questions about how they do their job. I find it better to reference a couple in order to get a more diverse and balanced perspective on a situation.* "

–Neurology nurse, St. Paul, MN

" *My classmates and I have tried to keep in touch so that we are mentoring each other. For a lot of new nurses, myself included, just having someone to talk to is a big help.* "

–Geriatric nurse, Oak Ridge, TN

" *Work where they have a new grad program. A mentor is very nice, but going through the process with other new grads is priceless.* "

–Rehabilitation nurse, Jaffrey, NH

SUCCESS STORIES

"I cried more than a couple times to my mentor when I felt like I didn't know anything, and he was really so encouraging. He made me the nurse I am today."

–Emergency room nurse, Santa Clarita, CA

"My charge nurse functions as my mentor. He is the best leader I have ever been around. He will drop anything he is doing if I have a question. He is also really supportive of me."

–Hospital staff nurse, Topeka, KS

"I found a mentor who is a mix of a drill sergeant and a sweet grandmother. She pushed me to be the best nurse I could be, but she was there to help and comfort when I messed up. Even though our personalities aren't exactly an ideal match, we have become close friends and trusting coworkers."

–Orthopedic nurse, Seabrook, TX

Whether or not you are successful in finding a mentor, you will still be faced with the challenge of developing yourself professionally once you begin your job. School made the structure of learning easy for you, as you progressed though a series of prearranged classes, each with a particular focus.

Now it is up to you to move forward on your own and choose your own focus. In the next chapter, experienced nurses share a wealth of tips on how to thrive and grow professionally in your working environment.

CHAPTER 10

Professional Growth

"*Every day is a new experience; a new day of learning and expanding professionally. I do not see an end to learning new things in many years to come. That's the beauty of nursing.*"

–Orthopedic nurse, Winona, MN

Once you graduate from nursing school, you might want to enjoy some freedom from the academic world of classes and grades. It's natural to feel like singing "No more teachers, no more books. . . ." But the reality is that the health-care field continues to change, and you need to keep up with the latest developments in nursing.

So take a deep breath—you have entered a lifelong learning zone. Not sure what a "lifelong learning zone" is? A learning timeline is waiting for you.

LEARNING TIMELINE

Activity 1

Read one professional journal or specialty nursing/health-care book. Start your first month on the job, and continue monthly thereafter forever.

Time Frame: It's very easy to procrastinate. Don't!

Activity 2

Participate in committees and task forces at your work or volunteer at a community organization. Keep this in mind your first three months on the job; get on board within your first year.

Time Frame: This is a great way to get to know people and enlarge your horizons beyond the limits of your current job.

Activity 3

Attend conferences or weekend workshops.

Time Frame: Although you probably won't go to a conference until after you've been on the job for a year, it never hurts to see what's out there right away.

Note: Plan ahead. You need time off and money in the bank (expenses may be reimbursed by your employer).

Activity 4

Study with continuing education courses or classes at a local college. By the end of your first three months on the job, make a list of which classes you want to take in the future. Then make your own timeline for when you want to take them.

Time Frame: Your state's requirements to renew your RN license will motivate you, but experiment freely!

ROOM FOR READING

To keep up-to-date on the latest happenings in health care, browse through a professional publication at least once a month. The easiest way to give your brain this regular intellectual jump start is to subscribe.

Then, when your journal arrives, just read the table of contents and mark which articles are most interesting.

If finances are an issue, get a discount on subscriptions by belonging to nursing organizations, or share the cost with your coworkers. Call the group a journal club and get together regularly to discuss a theme or article. Here are some journals that might be of interest:

American Journal of Nursing (AJN)

CIN: Computers, Informatics, Nursing

Clinical Journal of Oncology Nursing

Heart & Lung: The Journal of Acute and Critical Care

Holistic Nursing Practice

Image—The Journal of Nursing Scholarship (from Sigma Theta Tau)

International Honor Society of Nursing

JOGNN: Journal of Obstetric, Gynecologic, and Neonatal Nursing

Journal of Emergency Nursing

Journal of Pediatric Nursing

Journal of the American Psychiatric Nurses Association

Journal of Transcultural Nursing: A Forum for Cultural Competence in Healthcare Nursing

Pain Management Nursing

Pediatric Nursing

RN

PROFESSIONAL LITERACY

"Read nursing magazines so that you keep in touch with new ideas and trends in the field."

–Long-term-care nurse, Oak Ridge, TN

"Find the right reading material by asking for suggestions from older coworkers about what would help you in your job. They might also offer to lend you their copies."

–Dermatology nurse, Chicago, IL

"I found I really enjoyed taking the time to read the journals specifically for my area of nursing and trying to apply what I learned."

–Orthopedic nurse, Seabrook, TX

"*Open your mind: Read without limiting your topics.*"
–Public health nurse, Seattle, WA

CONTINUING EDUCATION

Your state board of nursing (BON) probably requires continuing education units (CEUs) when you renew your license. So, when you attend courses, make sure you get a certificate with the number of CEUs and the BON number of the course provider.

The insider advice is to keep those certificates forever. They are the nursing equivalent of gold! If you apply for a job, the certificates demonstrate acquired knowledge. This is crucial if you want to move to a new specialty. On the other hand, after taking a course in a particular field, you might find that the field doesn't appeal to you at all!

Now let's examine that gold. . . .

TIPS ON TAKING CLASSES

Always be open to attending seminars, even if they can only be scheduled on your day off.

–Cardiology nurse, Hampton, VA

Our hospital offers free continuing education classes as incentives for career growth and development. We also have an educational website where we can take free online classes during our days off.

–Psychiatric nurse, Elmendorf, TX

I get the class schedule of courses from the community college or local university. Even if I just take one class a year, I learn a lot. It expands my knowledge.

–Oncology nurse, Frederick, MD

CHOOSE A CONFERENCE

Attending your first conference as a working nurse is so exciting! Give yourself a target date of ending your first 100 days on the job knowing which event you want to attend. Not sure where to even begin? Here are some helpful tips:

- You don't need to rush. Conferences are usually organized years in advance, so you will have plenty of time to register and make travel arrangements. Just don't procrastinate.

- Find the conference that's right for you. Nursing publications are an excellent resource—they carry announcements and descriptions of upcoming conferences.

- Get your employer to help. Work out your time off with your supervisor well in advance and don't forget to ask if you'll be reimbursed by your employer.

- If finances seem problematic, consider attending a single day, or save on housing by staying with friends or family instead of at the hosting hotel. Or interest a colleague in going with you and share expenses. Yes, it will cost money . . . but you're worth it!

THE CAREER LIFT OF A CONFERENCE

Conferences are the perfect place to network. Below are some surefire tips for making sure you leave the event with the best contacts possible.

- Have a professional business card to bring to the conference; these can be produced fairly inexpensively either through your home computer and printer or at a local print shop. Business cards not only provide an excellent introduction your nursing qualifications but also demonstrate your interest in pursuing a business relationship. Your card should include contact information, certifications (RN, BSN, MSN), and a link to an online business profile or online resume.

- Arrive early. With only a small number of attendees present, you can start a lively conversation with a fellow "early bird."

- Get a list of attendees. If not provided at the outset, contact the check-in staff to see if they can make one available later. You might find the names of some people from your own organization whom you have not met before!

- Ask questions of speakers after their presentations. This gets you right in touch with experts in the field.

- If there are exhibits of equipment and supplies from vendors or health-care companies, check them out. Ask questions about their products and organizations. Enjoy their free literature.

- Study the agenda ahead of time so that you choose the most appealing lecture or panel presentations.

- Go to the poster sessions, in which space is provided for many presenters to do an informal stand-up show-and-tell about their work at the same time. Don't miss the opportunity to stroll through the area, check out the storyboards, and ask questions. It's very comfortable learning and networking.

- Invite other attendees to join you for your next meal. It's a great way to make new friends—and new contacts!

CONFERENCE CONDUCT

"*Go to conferences. It makes all the difference in the world when you have an active interest in your field. It makes you want to learn more.*"

—OB-GYN nurse, St. Louis, MO

" I have attended one conference each year for the past several years. Even when I didn't know a thing the first year, it was so inspiring to be with 6,000 other critical-care nurses. "

–Critical-care nurse, Los Gatos, CA

" When choosing a conference or workshop, don't narrow your scope of knowledge and/or practice to specialized areas. And don't always pick the clinical areas you are familiar with— experiment! "

–Operating room nurse, Barnesville, GA

COMMITTEE AND COMMUNITY INVOLVEMENT

Conferences tend to be big-time events requiring much preparation. On a smaller scale, you can get a career lift from your participation in teams that meet at work and in your community. The benefits are numerous:

"*Take on the challenge of getting involved in task forces that make changes in your department. You will be able to give input and be heard, and know how things get done.*"

–Emergency room nurse, Broken Arrow, OK

"*I volunteered for community organizations at the health department. This helped me to get to know people, because I relocated after graduation.*"

–Pediatric nurse, Danville, IL

"*We frequently participate in cancer/AIDS/heart walks as a team. It is good for developing a sense of unity.*"

–Critical-care nurse, Louisville, KY

YOUR OWN LEARNING RHYTHM

In addition to exploring unfamiliar outside sources for learning, you can find some wonderful educational opportunities right on the job. Take a look at the advice nurses have provided on the next few pages.

"*Not enough can be said for asking another nurse if you can watch or assist with a procedure that you have not done.*"

–Hospital staff nurse, Gwynn Oak, MD

"*In some cases, your supervisor or education department can provide you with some videos pertaining to the work you do.*"

–Medical-surgical nurse, St. Paul, MN

I took it upon myself to learn more about things that are very common on my floor, such as learning about often-used medications and understanding the reasons why doctors prescribe them. Sometimes meds aren't given for what the drug books say. I learned why the doctor prescribed them by reading the patients' charts thoroughly.

–Critical-care nurse, Newtown, PA

I ask myself why the physician has ordered labs, meds, etc., and then I take the time to find out.

–Cardiology nurse, Mamaroneck, NY

I concentrate on strengthening my skills that are weak by volunteering for the jobs that will give me more experience in those areas.

–OB-GYN nurse, Fort Riley, KS

"I allowed staffing to float me to other units to gain exposure to different kinds of nursing tasks and patient-care needs."

–Psychiatric nurse, Elmendorf, TX

"Hospitals will be more than happy to train you in many different areas, but you will probably have to be on call!"

–Critical-care nurse, North Highlands, CA

THE RENEWING COMMITMENT

"I think the first year is very tough on the new RN, but if you continue to keep learning, it will be easier in the future to learn new information."

–Neurology nurse, Albuquerque, NM

" I always consider there is room for improvement and accept constructive criticism. As long as your work is challenging, you will continue to grow professionally."

   –Long-term-care nurse, Martinez, CA

" Maintain your own personal goals. Participate in continuing education. Sit on professional committees and subscribe to professional journals. But in addition, participate in outside professional activities—volunteer and advocate for our profession."

   –OB-GYN nurse, Phoenix, AZ

Now that you've read about how to set in place a solid foundation for your professional growth, you might wonder, "How in the world am I ever going to take advantage of all those opportunities, and work, and still have time for a life? Isn't that asking for a lot of stress?"

You can expect that your early days in nursing will be hectic at times. And that's why in the next chapter, experienced nurses share with you their best advice on how to manage stress and achieve balance. Relax as you read on. . . .

CHAPTER 11

Keeping Energy Up and Stress Down

"*I have learned that there's nothing chocolate can't handle.*"
–Home-care nurse, Edinburg, TX

The bottom line is that nursing is an extremely stressful profession. But experienced nurses have found some creative ways to keep stress to a minimum without losing valuable time—or breaking their budgets. They have incorporated these methods of restoring their energy levels into their everyday work lives—and now they want to share them with you.

Some suggestions might seem obvious to you. But the fact is, many nurses are so busy nurturing others that they forget to take good care of themselves. Read this chapter on preventive methods and renewal techniques so that you remember!

BACK TO THE FUTURE

General exercise will develop your endurance for the workday. But there is one specific area of the body that nurses should target—the back. In fact, when nurses talk about lifting injuries or sore muscles, they refer to their condition as "having a nursing back." You should know how to keep your back in good shape right from the start.

Don't:

- Slump. Instead of curling up, stretch to an erect posture, and pull in your abdominal muscles as you lift your chest. (As a side benefit, this action can also make you appear taller and thinner!)

- Feel tied up in knots. Perform isometric exercises: Focus on a group of back or shoulder muscles, tense them as tightly as possible, and then relax them. Either way, you reestablish sensitive contact with your body.

- Lean forward when you lift something. That puts five times the pressure on your spine and back. Lift with your leg muscles instead.

- Move in two directions at once. Don't bend and twist, twist and reach, or bend and lift at the same time. Your body is not designed to handle those movements, and you are setting yourself up for injury.

TAKING CARE OF YOUR BODY

"Take three deep breaths and rotate your shoulders backward and forward. This will help relax your neck muscles."

–Neurology nurse, St. Paul, MN

> *"Get a back brace if you position patients in bed; pulling them up is harder than I ever thought it would be. Sometimes they feel like dead weight."*
>
> **–Cardiology nurse, Ellicott City, MD**

> *"Buy some inexpensive exercise bands and a wall chart that shows some simple stretches to limber up your tired muscles during your breaks."*
>
> **–Public health nurse, Milwaukee, WI**

EXERCISE YOUR JAW

Remember to focus on a shorter muscle group as well—your mouth! Conversation is key in keeping your stress levels down during the day. Here's what experienced nurses have to say on the subject:

"Try to take your break with someone else so you can share stories about how your day is going and laugh a little."

–Hospital staff nurse, Ontario, CA

"Going to the supervisor's office, closing the door, and venting does wonders!"

–Surgical nurse, Dubois, PA

BRAVO FOR BREAKS

Taking a short break that you have earned sounds like a simple no-brainer. But it's the most overlooked method of ensuring that you as a caregiver can refresh yourself to continue giving your best. Experienced nurses want to make sure that you incorporate breaks into your work routine from the start. They have different ways of saying it . . . but they want you to "Just do it!"

"*Don't be a martyr. Everyone needs to take time for breaks.*"

   –Critical-care nurse, Hamden, CT

"*Take breaks after a few hours of working so that you won't feel exhausted and worn out, because when emergencies arise, you'll need all the energy you have.*"

   –Psychiatric nurse, San Diego, CA

"*Time to regroup and reorganize. Sit in a quiet place off the floor and take slow, deep breaths. Relax and give yourself a pep talk, like, 'I'm going to go back and get things done and nothing is going to bother me. Now I'm wide awake and ready to go.' If you tell yourself that enough times, you will have a better attitude and feel more awake.*"

   –Critical-care nurse, Newtown, PA

"Go to the bathroom when you need to! Nurses are notorious for 'holding it!'"

–Medical-surgical nurse, Mt. Pleasant, SC

"Walking seems to be the trend for most staff nurses during their breaks. They walk briskly around the hospital premises and rest for a few minutes afterward before resuming their tasks. Some take naps for 30 minutes, especially if they work the graveyard shift."

–Psychiatric nurse, Elmendorf, TX

FOOD FOR THOUGHT

With all the running around you'll be doing, sometimes it will be hard to schedule your own meal times. All of a sudden, your usual eating time is long past and you're irritable and starving. How can you avoid this? See what experienced nurses advise that you do:

"Carry snacks in your pockets: raisins, crackers, etc. Set up a buddy system to take a lunch break. You watch some else's patients while she takes lunch and vice versa."

–Recovery room nurse, Owings Mills, MD

"I make sure that I have something with me that is quick and easy to eat, like some granola or an energy bar, so that if things get really hectic, I can still get a little bit of food in me."

–Pediatric nurse, Chicago, IL

"The lunchtime break is vital for me. I'm still on the unit and maintain responsibility for my patients during that time. But with my patients settled, when I sit down to eat, I can truly use that as a time for a little relaxation rather than worrying about the tasks that are still hanging over my head."

–Pediatric nurse, Baltimore, MD

"I try to stay well hydrated and eat enough protein before my shift to last me just in case I get a late lunch. The last thing anyone needs is a hypoglycemic nurse."

–Perioperative nurse, El Cerrito, CA

FEEDING THE SPIRIT

Increasingly, nurses are finding that nourishing the mind-body connection is important to achieving optimum health. Here's what some nurses add to their restoration repertoire:

"Get in touch with your spiritual side to keep centered."

–Urology nurse, Kalamazoo, MI

"Take a moment of silence between every patient."

–Cardiology nurse, Brooklyn, NY

"Keep a calendar and when you reach the one-, two-, and three-month anniversaries, circle the day. Congratulate yourself!"

–Ambulatory-care nurse, Milwaukee, WI

"If you have a performance evaluation scheduled, arrange to get a massage right afterward or go for a long walk—either as self-congratulations, or to de-stress!"

–Alternative-medicine nurse, Palo Alto, CA

THE ENVIRONMENT FOR RENEWAL

"Take a quick breath of fresh air once a day to clear your head. You need to have some relief from the constant 'hospital noise' in your ears."

–Cardiology nurse, Ellicott City, MD

"*Take advantage of your building's real stair-stepper. Take a quick five-minute trek up and down the stairs.*"

   –Critical-care nurse, Louisville, KY

"*Go to the restroom, lock the door, and take a breather. I go to the nursery right around the corner and look at the newborns.*"

   –Intensive care unit nurse, San Antonio, TX

"*Go to the cafeteria for lunch instead of staying in the department. The sounds of conversations and the aroma of different foods add to your sense of relaxation. And if you run into a friend, you'll both benefit.*"

   –Surgical nurse, Yuba City, CA

"Sit in a quiet room, even the supply closet, and relax for a minute. It's especially helpful when you have so much work that you don't even know where to start. When you leave, it's clear what needs to get done first, and how to proceed with the rest of your day."

–Pediatric nurse, Chicago, IL

"I have an aromatherapy highlighter. It's lavender-scented. I must look crazy smelling my highlighter, but it definitely helps me to de-stress and refocus."

–Telemetry nurse, Brick, NJ

Tip!

Your patients and their families are going to provide you with a lifetime of amazing learning experiences during you first 100 days. Get a blank journal that fits comfortably in your hands and use it like a diary to record the events that move you emotionally. Just as you would write a progress note, record the date and time. After all, it is a progress note—yours!

THE MENTAL HEALTH DAY

A time-honored tradition in nursing is taking a day off every once in a while. (The fact of the matter is, you're going to need it!) You should be alert to signs that you need such respite:

- Misplacing things that you need
- Getting to a place and not remembering what you came for
- Finding yourself overly critical of other people
- Feeling "run-down" or as though you are coming down with some illness
- Nightmares or insomnia
- Feeling like crying without knowing what triggered that feeling

TAKE TIME AWAY

"*Take a day off; don't overdo it. Overtime money is nice, but you are no good as a nurse if you're worn out.*"

–Critical-care nurse, Searcy, AR

"Don't take work home with you. Leave the stress and headaches behind."

—OB-GYN nurse, Point Pleasant, WV

"After work, forget everything, including the mistakes. Also, doing things outside your normal routine will refresh you."

—Public health nurse, Seattle, WA

ATTITUDE ADJUSTMENT

"Sometimes when I'm having an emotional day, I just try to remember that this too will pass."

—Home-care nurse, Center, TX

"Know that even the longest day has an end."

—OB-GYN nurse, Baltimore, MD

"I always try to remember to smile and laugh even when I am having a bad day. And if I am having a bad day, I try to remind myself that in order to truly appreciate the good days, everyone has to have a bad one every once in a while."

–Perioperative nurse, El Cerrito, CA

"I focus on the things I was able to accomplish in a timely manner that day and always try to keep a positive mind-set for my patients."

–OB-GYN nurse, Fort Riley, KS

Hopefully, reading about the de-stressing techniques in this chapter upped your relaxation level. The next chapter ups the smile factor: It spells out the perks of nursing. There are many ways nurses get rewarded—and a lot of them could only come from working in this special field.

CHAPTER 12

The Fun Perks of Nursing

"*I get to have as many Band-Aids as I want!*"
–Medical nurse, St. Catharine's, Ontario

Here's a fun fact for you: Perk is short for perquisite, the incidental benefits and advantages you get from your job, over and above your salary. Nursing has many fun perks, as nurses will share with you in this chapter. The special fringe benefits of nursing involve an enjoyment of tangible things, as nursing is a very down-to-earth profession, combined with the pleasure of heavy-duty contact with people.

BENEFICIAL BENEFITS

Each section in this chapter will impart a new perk that you will receive as a new nurse. Read on and enjoy!

"Tuition reimbursement means you get good training and have better advancement opportunities for free!"

–Oncology nurse, New York, NY

"We get a lot of vacation time—five weeks from the start—working for the government."

–Medical-surgical nurse, Summerville, SC

"The salaries are very competitive. Nursing is very much in demand these days, and after a couple of years of experience, the doors really open for you to be involved in a profession that's very monetarily rewarding."

–**Critical-care nurse, Chicago, IL**

"I really appreciate work bonus pay—huge hourly wages for any time done after your regular 36 hours."

–**OB-GYN nurse, Baltimore, MD**

FLEXIBILITY

"It's not always eight to five. I am not confined to a hospital unit or office setting all day."

–**Home-care nurse, Edinburg, TX**

I get to submit the schedule that I would like, and most of the time I get what I ask for. Also, I work twelve hour shifts, so I essentially work seven days out of fourteen.

–Intensive care unit nurse, Lynchburg, VA

You can work wherever you want—there are no boundaries.

–Hospital-staff nurse, Braintree, MA

I love taking off six days in a row without having to use vacation time.

–Critical-care nurse, Searcy, AR

Having weekdays off to run errands without rush-hour traffic or lines is fantastic.

–Intensive care unit nurse, Columbia, MD

FREEBIES

"*Nurses get free consultations from doctors that they work with.*"

–Critical-care nurse, Fayetteville, NC

"*Being a travel nurse means that I get free furnished housing.*"

–Orthopedic nurse, Philadelphia, PA

"*When surgery cases for the day are done, you get to go home early if you want.*"

–Surgical nurse, Yuba City, CA

"*We get a useful gift every May during Nurses' Week from our director of nursing.*"

–Hospital staff nurse, Milwaukee, WI

EXPERIENCES YOU DON'T GET ELSEWHERE

"Eating popcorn out of bedpans (unused). Hanging out with the 'colorful' people who show up in the ER at 2:00 A.M. on Saturday."

–Emergency department nurse, Henderson, KY

"Sometimes when we are without a counselor on the mental health unit, the nurses have the opportunity to conduct groups for the patients. My favorite is expressive arts, where the staff member conducting the group can participate as well."

–Psychiatric nurse, Greencastle, PA

"I love interacting with little ones or getting through to and developing a rapport with teenagers. I can also be more silly and lighthearted with children and their parents than I feel I can be with adults alone."

–Pediatric nurse, Chula Vista, CA

THE VARIETY OF EXPERIENCES

"You learn something new every day; it never becomes monotonous."

–Oncology nurse, Warminster, PA

"You interact and collaborate with lots of different people in different fields—pharmacy, nutrition, physical therapy, and respiratory therapy just to name a few!"

–Hospital staff nurse, Whispering Pines, NC

"You meet a lot of people from different walks of life, cultures, and traditions. You grow and your understanding also grows, and you become a better person."

–Psychiatric nurse, Elmendorf, TX

"You have unique relationships with people. Being a nurse bonds you very quickly with other nurses and also with patients."

   –Intensive care unit nurse, Columbia, MD

HONOR AND PRESTIGE

"I love having RN behind my name. I even wear my nametag to the grocery store."

   –Geriatric nurse, Helenwood, TN

"People treat me with a certain respect because I'm a nurse."

   –OB-GYN nurse, Philadelphia, PA

"Most patients recognize that it takes a very special personality to put up with the things nurses deal with every day."

   –Infertility clinic nurse, Mount Prospect, IL

APPRECIATION FROM PATIENTS

"*Getting a hug from a patient for just being there.*"

–**Geriatric nurse, Oak Ridge, TN**

"*Patients telling you how wonderful you are! Families bringing you goodies!*"

–**Surgical nurse, Winston-Salem, NC**

"*Seeing patients come back just to say 'Hi.'*"

–**Pediatric nurse, Fort Myers, FL**

"*Patients thank you for your kindness and ability to care. That may be the best perk.*"

–**Ear, nose, and throat nurse, Knoxville, TN**

MEANINGFUL WORK

"It is a pleasure to follow the patients I've taken care of as they recover or overcome their illness."

–Pediatric nurse, Baltimore, MD

"There's such a joy in taking great care of someone. Even though you're dead tired when you leave, you can feel as if you've accomplished a lot."

–Intensive care unit nurse, Atlanta, GA

"You will touch the hearts and leave a lasting impression on patients and families. You can't help but make a difference if you are good at your job."

–Critical-care nurse, Norridge, IL

"I am surrounded by the smartest and most compassionate people every day. My coworkers are always there for a good laugh. I only work three days a week. For working extra shifts, we earn gift certificates. And I make a difference in a person's life every day I come in to work. What I do really matters!"

–Hospital staff nurse, Topeka, KS

After hearing about the perks of being a nurse, the burning question is: Do they offset the challenges and possible downsides that experienced nurses shared with you in the previous chapters? Well, over a million nurses at work today in this country think so!

In previous chapters, you read about the best and the worst of what you might face . . . and how to enjoy and cope. In the next chapter, experienced nurses give you their final words of wisdom before you head out into the working world. They are totally supportive of you and want you to be a roaring success!

CHAPTER 13

Final Words of Wisdom

> "*Work with your heart. Every chance to learn, love, and be compassionate is a moment well spent.*"
>
> **—Long-term-care nurse, Winona, MN**

You are almost at the end of this book, but at the same time, you are at the beginning of an exciting and meaningful career. You have been given tips on how to deal with the day-to-day issues, cope with the best and worst of the people problems, renew your energy, and enjoy your well-earned rewards. What more can you ask for? Lots!

PARTING WISDOM

The hundreds of experienced nurses who contributed to this book want you to have their parting advice before you to launch your career.

HAVE PATIENCE

"*Give yourself a year to feel comfortable at your new job.*"

–Critical-care nurse, Westminster, CA

"*Pace yourself. Buy yourself some Advil, chocolate, and a good pair of comfortable shoes.*"

–Home-care nurse, Edinburg, TX

"*Don't be too hard on yourself. Allow room for growth. You will always be learning and will be often humbled. Just keep adding to your knowledge, and realize how much you have grown as you progress in your new job.*"

–Medical surgical nurse, St. Paul, MN

PERSEVERE

"*Don't expect to know everything right out of school—it takes time to learn the specific things about your unit. Don't get frustrated.*"

–Hospital staff nurse, Retsof, NY

"*No matter how rough things may seem, stick with it. Don't give up! It really does get better once you are over that initial learning curve.*"

–Medical-surgical nurse, Summerville, SC

"*Starting a new job can be intimidating. Be yourself, be confident, and relax. If someone gets to you, let it go. Hang in there.*"

–Operating room nurse, Gilliam, MO

BE CONFIDENT

"*Keep your chin up. You can do anything you set your mind to.*"

–Telemetry nurse, Georgetown, KY

"*Believe in yourself and your abilities. With each day that passes, you've gained that much more knowledge.*"

–OB-GYN nurse, Philadelphia, PA

"*Don't let anyone walk all over you. You have to be tough!*"

–Infertility clinic nurse, Kansas City, MO

REMEMBER YOU ARE NOT ALONE

"*Don't panic—others are always there to help if you don't know what to do.*"

–Hospital staff nurse, Boston, MA

"*Communicate with your coworkers. When people don't communicate, it can make the working environment very hostile. It makes such a difference when people talk to each other about things.*"

–Renal unit nurse, Leawood, KS

"*Don't lose contact with your nursing friends! Oftentimes, our significant others don't really know what we do every day and the stresses we experience, but our nursing friends do. Once a month, a group of us from our nursing school meet for lunch. We are there to laugh, have fun, tell stories, and support each other.*"

–OB-GYN nurse, Kansas City, MO

NEVER STOP LEARNING

"Always strive to learn new things. Be open to change. Don't lock yourself into one type of nursing."

–Critical-care nurse, Phoenixville, PA

"It's okay to not know. It's more than okay to ask."

–Hospital staff nurse, Baltimore, MD

"Don't be afraid to ask questions! It is better to be sure and risk feeling inadequate than to make a mistake. Most other nurses will be happy to answer your question, and your patients will be better off for it."

–Pediatric nurse, Chicago, IL

"Learn as much as you can and put all your effort into your job. You will get out of it as much as you put in."

–Hospital staff nurse, Baltimore, MD

FOLLOW THE RIGHT PATH

"Listen to your instincts. Don't let other people tell you 'It's okay' when you know it isn't. Stick to your ethics."

–Intensive care unit nurse, Columbia, MD

"In the unfortunate case of a lawsuit, documentation is so important. If you don't document everything you did for a patient, then in an attorney's eyes, it did not happen. You have to watch out for yourself. If you are not sure if you are documenting well, check with your supervisor or mentor. Have him review your notes."

–OB-GYN nurse, Chesapeake, VA

"Nursing is not just a profession but a vocation. You will never feel you have worked a day in your entire life if you love what you do."

–Allergy clinic nurse, Gardena, CA

KEEP EVERYTHING IN PERSPECTIVE

"Be self-sacrificing, but establish your boundaries to maintain your sanity."

–Nurse practitioner, Nashville, TN

"Your role as an RN is important—very important, and that will never change. But remember that you also need time to enjoy your own life outside of work or you will get burned out quickly and all too soon."

–Oncology nurse, Frederick, MD

"*You can't do it all. Worry only about the immediate task at hand. Don't bring your stress or job home; leave it in your locker.*"

–**Hospital staff nurse, Braintree, MA**

VALUE PATIENT CARE

"*Let your care be driven by your knowledge, softened by your compassion, and guided by your heart.*"

–**Perioperative nurse, El Cerrito, CA**

"*Nursing is one career where what you do may not be appreciated at that time, but once the patients are better, they remember you.*"

–**Home-care nurse, Edinburg, TX**

Communicate with your patients—let them know you are there for them if they have questions. And always keep your patients updated about their care. They really appreciate it and it lessens their anxiety, which in turn helps you better deal with them.

–Oncology nurse, Orlando, FL

Use common sense more than anything you learned in school. It's life, not the classroom.

–Critical-care nurse, Scranton, PA

Keep the patients number one. If you do that, then all the other conflicts with staff and other problems are minimal.

–Psychiatric nurse, Greencastle, PA

> " *I see more miracles and have more heartwarming experiences than I expected. Every day there is someone new who touches your heart.* "
>
> **–Critical-care nurse, Topeka, KS**

FIND YOUR NICHE

Of all the important messages that fill this book, one last one is critical. These days, the scope of what you can do as a nurse is so vast that you have many choices of where to contribute. Plus, additional nursing jobs that do not currently exist will be created in the years ahead.

In either a traditional setting or a nontraditional environment, there is a welcoming place, your very own niche, where your talents and enthusiasm will fit and be appreciated. It is up to you to not settle for second-best. Go for the gold!

RECOGNIZE YOUR CHOICES

"*Accept that you chose a career that isn't often a nine-to-five workday, and you knew that coming in. Whining doesn't make anyone's day any easier.*"

–Pediatric nurse, Baltimore, MD

"*There are many options for you in terms of the type of nursing you want to do. So if you are not happy with what you're doing, don't be afraid to take a chance to branch out to something different.*"

–Emergency department nurse, New York, NY

"*Know that you can always move from specialty to specialty. Nursing has freedom and a kind of power derived from experience.*"

–Cardiology nurse, Ellicott City, MD

FINDING YOUR FIT FEELS FANTASTIC!

When you discover your place in nursing, you enjoy the results the rest of your life! Nurses remember forever the moment they first found their niche:

> "*Being able to make it through a day and go home knowing I had been a part in helping save a life.*"
>
> **–Critical-care nurse, Searcy, AR**

> "*Organizing myself enough to get through the day, carrying out all orders, signing charts and documentation, and still be able to badge out at a reasonable time.*"
>
> **–Hospital staff nurse, Whispering Pines, NC**

"When I got through a day and didn't go home and question everything I did in my head."

–Recovery room nurse, Martinez, CA

"Realizing that I was going to survive and what seemed so impossible while in school, or on my first day, was happening. I will be successful."

–Orthopedic nurse, Philadelphia, PA

The ABCs of Success!

When all is said and done, only you will know when you've made the rite of passage from a new graduate to an established nurse (and hopefully this book will have helped you get there!). Since the scope of nursing activities is so broad, experienced nurses each have a unique sense of that defining moment—of that breakthrough achievement during their first 100 days. Here are their A to Zs of success. One day soon, you'll be able to add yours to the list!

"*Assisting a surgeon as a scrub nurse in a major surgery.*"
–Operating room nurse

"Being able to help others heal."
  –Pediatric nurse

"Caring for all my patients like they are my own family."
  –Psychiatric nurse

"Developing a good relationship with the care team."
  –Critical-care nurse

"Experiencing the first day I went to do something and didn't say, 'Where is my nursing instructor?'"
  –Medical-surgical nurse

"Finding someone in respiratory distress and reversing it. To this day, when in the hospital, this patient calls me her angel. She tells everyone I saved her life!"

–Telemetry nurse

"Getting organized in the morning, having everything written down, and getting the big picture."

–Intensive care unit nurse

"Having a patient call me on the phone at work after his discharge to tell me that he'd always love me for the excellent way I cared for him after his heart surgery."

–Critical-care nurse

"*Inserting a nasogastric tube into a pediatric patient and acting confident in performing this task without the patient knowing I was a nervous wreck on the inside.*"

–Pediatric nurse

"*Juggling a minimum of six patients.*"

–Pediatric nurse

"*Knowing I was a productive part of my health-care team.*"

–Surgical nurse

"*Learning to ask questions when I was not sure of something instead of thinking that I should already know it.*"

–Telemetry nurse

"*Making a difference in the lives of families with sick babies.*"
   –**Pediatric nurse**

"*Noticing subtle changes in a patient's condition that may have led to something more dangerous.*"
   –**Cardiology nurse**

"*Overcoming my fear of physicians. I realized that they are humans, too!*"
   –**Emergency room nurse**

"*Passing meds and finishing charting by the time the shift was over.*"
   –**Orthopedic nurse**

"*Q*uestioning a doctor who wanted to discharge an unstable patient. I stood up for the patient."

–Trauma/surgical nurse

"*R*unning my first Code Blue for a cardiac arrest and having a doctor who is known for not having good people skills tell me I did a wonderful job."

–Critical-care nurse

"*S*tarting an IV on my own was definitely a high point."
–Hospital staff nurse

"*T*eaching a patient who agreed to make life-changing decisions."
–Organ procurement nurse

"*Understanding that I am empowered every day by what I do and wanting to continue in it.*"

   –Critical-care nurse

"*Valuing the day that I realized that I can be a great nurse; compliments from coworkers really help to boost one's ego.*"

   –Step-down unit nurse

"*Wanting to continue in nursing, being energized every day by what I do.*"

   –Critical-care nurse

"*Xeroxing a copy of my advanced cardiac life-saving certificate for my files. I remember thinking it was going to be awful to go through—but it really wasn't!*"

   –Critical-care nurse

"*Yielding to my gut instinct. Now I trust it.*"
   –Hospital staff nurse

"*Zeroing in on why I became a nurse: to help those who cannot help themselves.*"
   –Telemetry nurse